T0186913

Cause of Death

Cause of Death

Dr Geoffrey Garrett
and Andrew Nott

ROBINSON

ROBINSON

First published in Great Britain in 2001 by Robinson,

Copyright © Geoffrey Garrett and Andrew Nott 2001

11

The moral right of the authors has been asserted.

All rights reserved.
No part of this publication may be reproduced, stored in a retrieval
system, or transmitted, in any form, or by any means, without the prior
permission in writing of the publisher, nor be otherwise circulated
in any form of binding or cover other than that in which it is published
and without a similar condition including this condition being
imposed on the subsequent purchaser.

A CIP catalogue record for this book
is available from the British Library.

ISBN: 978-1-84119-295-6 (paperback)
ISBN: 978-1-47210-804-3 (ebook)

Printed and bound by CPI Group (UK) Ltd, Croydon, CR0 4YY

Papers used by Robinson are from well-managed forests
and other responsible sources

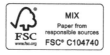

Robinson
An imprint of
Little, Brown Book Group
Carmelite House
50 Victoria Embankment
London EC4Y 0DZ

An Hachette UK Company
www.hachette.co.uk

www.littlebrown.co.uk

Contents

	List of Illustrations	vi
	Prologue	vii
	Introduction	1
1	The Devils in Disguise	9
2	A Savage Breeze	29
3	Mother Mac's	43
4	Mr Asia	79
5	Death as a Way of Life	93
6	The Police	107
7	Mad or Bad?	131
8	To Have or Have Not	151
9	The Moss	161
10	The Irish Connection	193
11	An Appealing Man	199
12	Man's Inhumanity to Woman	215
13	Cold and Steel	235
14	In Black and White	255
15	Unsolicited Male	265
16	Heat	281
17	Under Age	299
18	Making Faces	311
19	The Empty Sport	319
20	The Lord of Strangeways	325
	Index	335

List of Illustrations

The holdall used to hide Christine Marsh's body
The hammer used to kill Christine Marsh
Pauline Reade's white stiletto shoe
The passenger map of the doomed Manchester airport flight
The aftermath of the disaster†
The storeroom at Mother Mac's where the pyre of bodies was found
X-ray of Marty Johnstone's severed hand
Louise Brown*
Inspector Ray Codling*
PC John Egerton*
The discovery of skeletal remains in a shallow grave
The recovered pieces of the skeleton
DIY abortion kits
Dr Geoffrey Garrett at work

Tony Johnson*
An X-ray of Samuel McDougall's brain
The house outside which Christopher Downey was shot dead
An X-ray of Christopher Downey's thigh
Amanda Jane Allman*
An X-ray of Tahir Akram's head
Susan Hockenhull†
Ian Jebb's body being removed†
A tent showing the location of Susan Hockenhull's body†
The Summerland fire†
The Woolworth's fire*
Stages of the re-creation of Sabbir Kilu's face
Alan Lord on the roof of Strangeways jail*

† PA
* MEN Syndication
All other images are authors' own

Prologue

My first body came, appropriately, in a bag.

It was a green tartan canvas holdall less than two feet long, which might normally have carried a change of clothes, another pair of shoes, a spare shirt or two, a paperback book. Sandwiches.

In every sense it was an ordinary bag. Nothing about it would have attracted attention. No one would have had reason to wonder what it contained.

Murder, with its accompaniments of pain, anguish, sadness, fear and regret had, as usual, materialized in the most unassuming and commonplace manner.

The bag had unmistakable dried brown bloodstains on the zip and the handle. It was being cradled in the strong arms of a burly detective called Joe Mounsey, the head of Lancashire CID.

He'd telephoned me at Oldham Royal Infirmary and asked if I would meet him at Urmston Police Station, twelve miles away. I got in my old Jag and set off immediately.

For reasons never fully explained, murder victims tend to be found in the middle of the night or at a time that interrupts lunch. This was a lunchtime case and, although it was long ago, in October 1968, I recall that the meal I missed was steak and chips. It was a Thursday and in those days the

Infirmary canteen always served steak on Thursdays.

I had just been appointed Home Office pathologist with responsibility for assisting police inquiries when foul play is suspected and this was my first call-out in that capacity. I was already a consultant pathologist, working daily at the hospital, so corpses were nothing new to me. But this one, my first with the police, was always going to be special, important.

She was a seven-year-old schoolgirl.

When I arrived at the station Detective Chief Superintendent Mounsey spoke with me briefly, explaining that there was a body in the bag and asking how I wanted to proceed. We took the bag, unopened, to the nearest mortuary at Park Hospital, Davyhulme. There we were greeted by a group of nervous-looking CID trainees whose boss had given them the unwelcome news that this was the day they were going to get around to viewing a murder-case autopsy.

No one fainted, no one threw up and no one, apart from my assistant and I, said anything. For our own reasons we were all on edge. But the young officers all remained stoic, concentrating on controlling their stomachs while I tried to appear the calm, unruffled doctor used to all this and perfectly in command.

As I opened the bag it was as quiet as the grave.

The holdall sat, no doubt looking menacing to the trainees, on the mortuary slab, the shape inside pressing against the canvas but unrecognizable. Then I pulled gently but firmly at the zip. It clicked loudly as each metal tooth came undone.

Christine Marsh was lying inside, curled up, her head facing away from the fastening and her back uppermost. As with so many dead children, her body gave the immediate impression of being simply asleep.

No matter what logic tells you, no matter what you know for sure, the sight of a dead child is always more difficult to accept than the sight of a dead adult. There is that foolish, practically subconscious twinge of impossible hope that begs, ridiculously, *Let her wake.*

Christine Marsh was fully dressed in a grey coat, grey dress, red jumper, underslip, vest and red knickers. The clothes had not been disturbed. She wore red stockings but no shoes. I found one shoe in the bag once I had lifted her out. She wore a gold chain and her blonde hair was in a ponytail.

It is rarely useful or wise for a pathologist to consider how a person might have been while they were alive. Had this child once been bright-eyed, or coy and shy? Lively or quiet? Popular or difficult? Charming or devious? A loner or the leader of her young pack?

I could answer none of these questions. In life the child had been unknown to me and in death I would learn only those things that would be of use to the detectives. To try to think of what she had once been might be a distraction, a confusion. I could not concentrate on what once had been, merely on what was in front of me now.

I was not working on Christine Marsh, I was working on what had been left behind. My inquiries had nothing to do with the person people had known and my findings would be of no use to those who had laughed and played with her. Those who had loved her, who had shared her in life, would have little use for what I could tell them about her death. Mounsey, however, would.

Christine Marsh had been hit five times on the head with

a heavy object, probably a hammer. Three blows had left marks to the front and two others were obvious to the side. Her skull had suffered several fractures, causing brain damage. Apart from the head wounds she was a normal, healthy girl, so the cause of death was clear.

Mounsey was satisfied. The bag had been found in a neighbour's house, stuffed in a bedding box. The girl had apparently been talkative and inquisitive in life and had visited the neighbour while he was carrying out repairs to the bodywork of his car. She had asked one question too many – he had lost his temper, killed her with his panel-beater's hammer and hidden her body.

His eventual confession was believed because it matched the evidence provided by forensic scientists and by me. Blood samples collected at the autopsy matched those found on the hammer and in his car and his own description of the way he had attacked the little girl corresponded with my own findings.

He got life.

Since that day in 1968 1 have conducted autopsies in criminal investigations on 1,638 people, 104 of have been children. It is always the children who get to you. Every time, behind the cold, professional exterior, you can't help but think: *Oh no, not another child.*

Sooner or later I get to know something about the tragedy that surrounds each death. Sometimes the story is one of such misery that it cannot help but reach out to your innermost feelings and grip painfully. There have been several that, for various reasons, I still remember with genuine emotion rather than with just my analytical memory. There are others so horrible that I would love to be able to forget them.

But the job is sufficiently complex and, I believe, important for me always to approach it with as much detachment and professional control as possible.

The gruesome aspect is actually not too difficult to cope with – most of the time. Policemen, ambulance crews, firemen, everyone who works in medicine, all of them have to deal with death and injury. You cope because otherwise you can't function. It is required.

What happened in life to the child, the mother, the grandfather, the brothers and sisters before that life left them was never my concern. They came to me only after they had lost that force that caused their hearts to beat, their lungs to breathe, their brains to think; that caused them to live.

I was there for the cause of death.

Introduction

It would be useful before you read the following chapters for you to understand some principles of the post-mortem examination.

It would be surprising if you were not somewhat wary of the dead. Most people are. So allow me to make you feel, if not more at home amongst them, then at least more at ease through being better informed.

This book chronicles the story of my professional life over nearly forty years. During this time I spent many of my working hours performing autopsies on the recently – and, occasionally, not-so-recently – deceased.

While each case is unique, the methods and procedures used to unlock the secrets of the dead tend to be quite similar. So, to avoid unnecessary repetition and to assist your understanding, I would like to outline here some of the detail of how a post-mortem is conducted.

When crime was suspected, as it was in most of the cases in this book, my work usually began well away from the mortuary.

Often in a suspicious-death inquiry the most crucial segment is the first – at the crime scene itself. In the old days, policemen's boots too often trampled all around a body as detectives tried to look businesslike. But now, with forensic science capable of unearthing clues from the most apparently unpromising of situations, crime scenes are always sealed either immediately or at the earliest possible opportunity. I was one of the few people allowed past the blue tape.

It may be several hours after a body's discovery before it is moved. This is to ensure as far as possible the preservation of tell-tale signs that might later prove invaluable: it is sometimes simply necessary to wait until daylight to have a proper look. While this may seem to some to be less than dignified, the honest truth is that the dead don't mind. In these circumstances, they are, after all, the people who matter most.

The prime considerations for me at this stage are the position of the body and any piece or pieces of the body that may have become detached. This would include any body parts, body tissues or blood. Their distance from the body, their shape, the trajectory and direction of their separation are all important in assessing what has gone on.

On one occasion, the police were almost apologetic about calling me out to what they considered was surely an accident where an elderly man had tripped on his landing at home, fallen and hit his head with fatal consequences. On my arrival I was able to inform them that a murder had indeed taken place because I recognized a blob of grey mess adhering to the base of a wall a few feet from the corpse as brain matter. You don't get that kind of injury just by falling over.

However, on another case I noted that there were red stains on a wall next to the body of the victim and asked for samples to be taken. Forensic examination revealed they had been caused by the spillage of a can of fizzy blackcurrant cordial. The stains played no further part in the investigation.

The main evidence at this stage is photographic, backed up by meticulously made scale plans of the scene and diagrams of the body and any apparently relevant articles. All these tasks must be carried out with the body untouched and *in situ*.

I take the temperature of the body and check the ambient temperature of where it was found – which might be in a house, in a field, by a roadside, anywhere. This helps in trying to establish the time of death.

When everyone is satisfied that the initial parts of the inquiry have been completed, plastic bags are placed on the hands and over the head of the body and tied snugly. The whole body is wrapped in a plastic sheet and then placed in a body bag before being taken to the mortuary. The mortician there will always be alerted that a body is on its way but he will know no more until it arrives.

The body is first weighed and measured and then, before the body, the plastic sheet is examined. I have known bullets to drop out of a corpse during the bumpy ride to the mortuary, so the sheet is there to catch such items rather than allow any evidence to vanish. Any object found on the sheet is bagged, sealed and marked with identification labelling.

Similarly the bags on the hands and head of the body are removed and examined. The head, with its orifices and hair, and the hands, because of their natural function, are the most likely places where other bits of important material – sometimes very small – may be found. Also, at this stage, before any clothing is removed, samples of plucked and combed head-hair are taken, together with cuttings from the fingernails. The plucked hair includes the root, which can be used for DNA and drug analysis, while the combed hair and nails are checked for any fragments or residues that might prove useful.

The clothed whole corpse is examined in great detail in an attempt to locate any foreign body such as paint, pieces of wood, grass, dust, soil – anything at all. We have no idea at this stage what we are looking for so everything is bagged, sealed and labelled.

On one occasion a tiny smear of paint on the clothing of a road accident victim was later matched to a car, so providing good evidence that this was the vehicle responsible for the injuries that led to the individual's death.

In the past it was normal to take a sample of the aqueous humour from the eyes. The level of potassium found in this liquid rises in a straight line following death and proved quite an accurate measure of the time of death on many of my earlier autopsies. Later, however, it became a less popular procedure. Also it was a method that could not be used if there had been a serious head injury as the eyes were often damaged in such cases.

The clothing is removed slowly, layer by layer, and again carefully examined with photographs taken if necessary at each stage. Holes, marks, discolourations, scrapes and tears in the material are noted, later to be compared with any wounds on the body.

The naked body is then examined in great detail. Further hair samples are taken from the eyebrows and pubic area, while swabs are taken from the mouth, anus, genitalia and from any other exudates (apparent bodily fluids) that are discovered. While the swabs are being taken the relevant orifices are examined. Bruises and lacerations may be present in any or several of them.

Every inch of the skin – including that covering the hands and feet – is carefully checked for any injury, bruise, scar or injection mark. One time I found pinprick marks on the feet of a male nurse who had been injecting himself there. This was important evidence that could easily have been missed.

The hair surrounding any head injury is shaved. All wounds on the body are carefully measured, both in their extent and depth and also in relation to a fixed point on the body to provide as precise a position as possible. For instance, a stab wound to the chest could be described as being fifty-two inches from the ankle and three inches to the left of the midline. Accuracy can be critical in a courtroom situation.

It is vital that no area of skin is missed and no assumptions made too early. One woman found dead in a fire had burns consistent with her having been killed in a blaze on the front of her body. But when we turned her over we discovered that she had been stabbed numerous times in the back.

Further body-temperature readings are taken during this period and note is made of the degree of rigor mortis and body staining (due to the natural process of putrefaction). Again, all this assists with establishing a time of death.

It is only after all that work has been completed that dissection can begin.

My instruments are few but very sharp. They are made by a specialist firm in Whitechapel, London, coincidentally the hang-out in Queen Victoria's time of the killer known as Jack the Ripper, undoubtedly the most famous exponent of the criminal usage of such surgical equipment.

I can get by with a sharp scalpel, forceps, a pair of blunt-nose scissors, a pair of small coronary artery scissors, a brain-knife, a saw, a power saw, a ruler and probes.

The brain-knife is a long-bladed knife so-called because it is used to cut the brain into slices or sections before it is microscopically examined. However, this knife can be used to cut up any organ. The saws are for the bones, the skull in particular. The blunt-ended scissors limit the risk of my slicing through something I shouldn't while I am dissecting, especially when working in an area of densely compacted soft tissue such as the intestines.

The initial incision is dictated to some extent by the position of any injuries. But in most cases, and certainly in all standard forensic examinations, a Y-shaped incision is made that begins with cuts behind each ear that descend at an approximate forty-five-degree angle along the neck, meet at the top of the chest and then descend vertically as one to the pelvis.

Some practitioners, mostly in America, prefer to make their initial incision on a horizontal line across the top of the shoulders as it is less disfiguring. However, the Y shape allows a much better display of the larynx and makes the procedure of pulling back the skin of the face over the skull far less complicated. Consequently it is easier to demonstrate jaw fractures and other facial injuries.

The essential requirements for effective dissection are good lighting and sharp knives. All the knives have to have disposable blades because they blunt quickly and require changing regularly. There is a lot of tough tissue in a body and, unlike a roast leg of lamb, it has not been softened by cooking. Not usually.

The organs can be removed in blocks – it is sometimes easier to take out two or more in one go, the heart and lungs, for instance – but circumstances vary according to the situation.

If there are bullet or knife wounds that need tracing, then X-rays must be taken. This is vital in the case of bullets as they can do strange things inside a body, depending on which tissues and bones they hit and their muzzle velocity. For example, the first shot that penetrated one of my earlier subjects, Christopher Downey, of whom you will read more later, entered a buttock and was deflected by part of the pelvic bone down to the marrow cavity of the thigh bone.

During the internal examination, further examples of blood, urine, stomach contents and organs are taken for detailed forensic examination. Again, all are bagged, sealed and signed.

For obvious reasons, my report was always prepared as quickly after the examination as possible.

The work is, by its very nature, a long and sometimes rather messy procedure that offends all the senses, most significantly those of sight and smell. But I always felt that all the unpleasantness that others often brought to my attention was outweighed every time by the job's sheer fascination.

Now, if you will bear all that in mind, we will not need to waste time going through it all again.

I would like to welcome you to my mortuary. And I shall begin.

1

The Devils in Disguise

By the time Pauline Reade came to my table she had been dead for twenty-four years.

At the age of sixteen, on what had been a pleasant, fine July evening in 1963, she had persuaded her parents that she was quite capable, thank you very much, of walking to a local dance on her own.

Her girlfriend, who would normally have walked with her, had opted to go to the local cinema instead. But it was Friday night, Pauline had a new pink-and-gold dance outfit to show off and, anyway, the dance was only 400 yards down the road.

Like all decent mums and dads, Amos and Joan Reade were protective of their daughter and still saw her as a little girl, *their* little girl, their pride and joy. They would have preferred it if she'd been accompanied and they could have insisted, could have put their foot down. But the 1960s were in full swing and kids were rebelling. Flower Power bemused the older generations, rock and roll was here to stay and the post-war babies were becoming teenagers who were like no teenagers ever before.

Luckily for Amos and Joan, their Pauline had her feet firmly on the ground and, as they say, she knew a thing or two. She wouldn't do anything silly or take any daft risks. It was only her third visit to a 'hop' and she'd only ever come home late one time before, stepping sheepishly through the door at midnight. That time she had flung her arms around her mother who had been so worried and promised faithfully she'd never do it again.

Pauline was a convent-educated girl who went to Mass every Sunday and she wouldn't break her word. And, for goodness' sake, she was nearly a woman.

In truth, the result of the argument between the young lady and her doting folks was never much in doubt. Like a million other parents before and since, the Reades took another step towards the inevitable acceptance of their daughter's disappearing childhood and told her: 'OK, you can go. But be careful.'

Jauntily, another moral victory under her belt, feeling quite the bee's knees in her new 'grown-up' black blouse and gaily patterned skirt, Pauline began the five-minute journey from her small, neat, terraced home in Wiles Street, Gorton, Manchester, to the dance at the Railway Workers Social Club.

She never made it.

It was the year of the Profumo Affair, Harold Macmillan had just resigned as Prime Minister and John F. Kennedy was the charismatic, adored US President, five months short of his own terrible date with destiny. But, rightly, none of this would have been the concern of the likeable working-class lass who was a trainee confectioner at the local factory where her dad also worked. Her young head was full instead with thoughts of boys and The Twist, and as she walked she would have whistled the tunes from that week's BBC Hit Parade, stepping in time to the rhythms in her head, her fingers clicking. Gerry and the Pacemakers were Number One with 'I Like It' and 'It's My Party' by Lesley

Gore was up there too. The Beatles' latest was just ahead of Elvis Presley's 'Devil In Disguise'.

Then, in the bright sunlight of an early evening in summer, as Pauline strolled along without a care in the world, someone spoke her name.

A rather battered van had pulled up and, leaning out of the open driver's window, a woman she knew reasonably well, the sister of a girl called Maureen who lived next door but one, called her over. It would not have occurred to Pauline that there was anything to worry about. There was no reason to check the street to see if there were other people around, no point in panicking that the street was deserted apart from her and this acquaintance beckoning her closer. No need to run.

The trusting youngster would have smiled her naturally wide smile and walked towards the van to see what the woman wanted. Pauline liked to pass the time of day and chat.

From behind the steering wheel, the driver, Myra, who looked older than her twenty years with her dyed blonde hair, put on her friendliest tone and made the younger girl an offer she couldn't refuse. The persuasive, tempting lies dripped off her tongue like grease. It was like taking candy from a baby. Easy meat.

Plausibly, she explained how she had lost an expensive pair of gloves and needed Pauline's help to search for them. If the girl agreed, the woman offered, she'd reward her with pop records. A pile of discs was stacked invitingly on view in the back of the van.

Now, nothing was going to stop Pauline going to the dance: she'd been looking forward to it too much. But it was only 7:30 in the evening and there'd be plenty of time to go looking for the gloves and then come back and still make a night of it. And some of the records looked great. As she climbed willingly into the passenger side, she probably thought: *This is my lucky day!*

In subsequent interviews, Myra Hindley always insisted that Pauline didn't give her any problems in the van, although Saddleworth Moor was a good thirty to forty minutes' drive away. It would have been a reasonable assumption that, as they got further and further away from the dance hall, the younger girl would have become a little nervous, a touch suspicious, fearful, if nothing else, of missing out on her big night. But no, said Hindley, she was no trouble, no problem.

They would have arrived at the desolate, empty moor shortly before 8.30 p.m., the summer evening light still good. Hindley stopped, applied the handbrake and got out, saying: 'This is it.' By the killer's own account, even when they were joined a short time later by her boyfriend, Ian Brady, Pauline sensed nothing amiss. She went quietly onto the moor.

Amos and Joan Reade never saw their daughter again, alive or dead. They neither needed nor wanted to see what was left when, in 1987, her body was finally exhumed from its makeshift tomb. They buried Pauline in consecrated ground at Gorton cemetery, relieved that after twenty-four years they could at last grieve and weep for their child and bury with her mortal remains any lingering false hopes that she would walk through their door and apologize for being late.

We learned quite a lot about what happened to Pauline in the hours when she was at the mercy of the Moors Murderers, those last hours of her life. But the passage of so much time had removed too many of the clues, the tell-tales, the signs that we rely on in forensic medicine so that the full details of what she went through were beyond our skills to uncover. Perhaps it was as well.

In November 1963, five months after Pauline's death, twelve-year-old John Kilbride vanished. Seven months after that another twelve-year-old, a gap-toothed mite called Keith Bennett, disappeared without trace. On Boxing Day 1964 it was the turn of ten-year-old Lesley Ann Downey. Finally, Edward Evans, aged seventeen, was hacked to death at a house in Hattersley. A horrified witness to that carnage told police what had happened in a frantic, terrified phone call and Hindley and Brady, still in the house with the corpse, were arrested.

A trail led detectives to the moor where they discovered the bodies of Lesley Ann Downey and John Kilbride. Soon 'Moors Murderers' became the most infamous phrase in British criminal history.

Both of them were sentenced to life, Brady on all three counts, Hindley for the murders of Evans and Lesley Ann Downey, with a further seven years for harbouring her boyfriend after he had killed John Kilbride.

It was twenty years later before there was any hard evidence to link Brady and Hindley to the disappearances of Pauline Reade and Keith Bennett. Then renewed Press speculation about a connection to 'other murders' led the then head of Greater Manchester CID, Chief Super-intendent Peter Topping, to open the inquiry once more.

I was one of the first people Topping told of his intentions since he would require my involvement if he discovered any human remains. At the time I thought he had no chance of finding anything and if he had sought my advice I would have told him not to bother. Today, despite the discovery of Pauline's body, I am still not sure it was the right move.

This was a case that had refused to go away for a number of reasons. It had undoubtedly been the most notorious murder trial ever conducted in this country. Sure, there have been people who have carried out killings of even greater savagery and there are individuals who have claimed far more victims than Brady and Hindley. But if you asked ten members of the public to name just one famous British murder, nine would choose The Moors Murders.

Most of all, it was Myra's involvement that fixed the horror in the minds of every parent in Britain. A woman had abducted children to kill them for pleasure. A woman! In the 1960s this was, as the title of the famous book had it, beyond belief. This genuinely shocking realization did not just *touch* a nerve with the public at large, it wrenched it out by the roots.

Then, of course, there was the tape. Hindley and Brady made the recording while they did what they did to little Lesley Ann who, in her photograph, looked as delicate and vulnerable as porcelain. Its playing in court at Chester Assizes, as she begged for mercy, was one of the most harrowing sounds – and the most damning evidence – ever heard in a courtroom.

The toughest policemen who, until then, had thought they'd seen it all, went home and cried for hours. Experienced crime reporters who had been briefed and knew what was coming returned to their families badly shaken and hugged their own children until the kids asked them to stop. The general public was aghast.

There was not the faintest doubt after the jury heard the

tape that the pair would be convicted. From this point on, during a period when tabloid journalism became more and more lurid in this country, it was inevitable that every time a small piece of gossip about Hindley or Brady was aired it would make headlines. When either killer said or did anything, however inconsequential, it made the Press, and when high-profile figures, notably Lord Longford, tried to intervene on behalf of the pair, it was a front-page story.

Although they were safely locked away, the Moors Murderers remained news. Another reason why news editors wouldn't let the story go was that they, along with the police, were convinced that the evil pair had also claimed the lives of the two youngsters who had not been found on the moor but who had vanished in similar circumstances to Lesley Ann Downey and John Kilbride.

Over the years there were occasional references, veiled suggestions and periodic hints in the papers that all had not yet been revealed. The couple were also a good target for such speculation because it was unlikely they would sue. How, after all, could Hindley and Brady claim that their good names were being blackened by Press innuendo or speculation?

Also, although Brady, declared insane and enjoying solitude in the secure Ashworth Hospital, Merseyside, always said he did not want to be released, Hindley courted the media from Cookham Wood prison and apparently enjoyed the publicity.

In the middle 1980s conjecture reached its zenith and Detective Chief Superintendent Topping decided the time was right to get involved. When he told me what he had planned I thought he was wrong, essentially since I thought he would fail. The moor is huge and children are small. It *is* possible for bodies to survive intact over a long period of time but this is quite rare. Of the bodies of the two children found quickly, Lesley Ann Downey's, found in preserving peat, like Pauline's, was in good condition, but little was left of that of John Kilbride, buried in a stream bed.

The other point was that the murderers were already in prison and, due to the pressure of practically unanimous public opinion, were unlikely to be coming out. They were, in effect, doing time for all their crimes.

The search, I thought, would kindle hope in the families of these long-dead youngsters that was unlikely to be realized. They had suffered so dreadfully over the years: would any new inquiry do much more than bring back all that pressure and sadness and remind them of their loss without providing anything substantial to fill the space? Would it, indeed, do more harm than good?

In the event, Pauline's family *did* go through fresh suffering. But they expressed their deep gratitude to Topping for providing finally the opportunity to pay their last respects to a loved one taken so abruptly from their midst. It seems that, to them, the recovery of their child's body was worth the cost.

Winnie Johnson, the mother of Keith Bennett, the twelve-year-old boy whose body was not found but is now also known with certainty to be a murder victim buried somewhere on the moor, has consistently praised the now-retired policeman for his efforts despite his eventual failure to locate her son's remains. She still visits the moor regularly, occasionally with a shovel.

Topping said in his autobiography that both Hindley and Brady had confessed to him, in the presence of lawyers, their parts in the two killings. Neither has since denied this allegation. The case, however, is not completely closed. There was a finding of 'unlawful killing' at the inquest into the death of Pauline Reade, but the hearing did not name the killers and the then Director of Public Prosecutions, Alan Green QC, decided it was not in the public interest for either of them to face further murder charges.

I feel, despite this confirmation of the fate of the youngsters, that the merits of the investigation are still open to debate. Topping said that he agreed with Green's decision not to prosecute. But, if a detective's final goal is not a prosecution, what is it? If all his efforts do not result in the country being made a safer place, is he not taking upon himself the wrong task? He did well to discover what he did – it was in many ways a triumph – but was he tilting at windmills?

A team of experienced (and expensive) detectives, including the most senior operational detective in Manchester (Topping himself), spent months wielding spades to solve crimes that, perhaps, did not really need solving. There was, for all practical purposes, no doubt in anyone's mind what had befallen Pauline and Keith: they had died at the hands of Hindley and Brady.

However, once Topping started, the pressure of publicity was so powerful that it would have been extremely difficult, even if he had wanted, for him to have called a halt. Having spent hours interviewing both Hindley and Brady he knew considerably more than he was telling and, bolstered by this secret insight, he took criticism on the chin, biding his time, giving little or nothing away.

He was genuinely confident that what he had learned from them would lead him to his goal. However, particularly as the inquiry dragged on for weeks without any significant result, Topping's insistence on keeping to himself the reasons why he was so confident led to much speculation about how the operation was being handled. This grated with a man so used to dealing with cold facts, but he steadfastly kept his own counsel.

Hindley and Brady had both confessed to him their involvement in the murders of this boy and girl and had given him details of where the bodies were buried. In time, both killers visited the moor amid massive publicity to point out sites that they claimed could be the places where their victims lay. It is still unclear whether they were making genuine efforts to assist the search or were playing yet another morbid game, relishing the rekindled pain of the families and what was, up until then, the failure of the police.

Their confessions were in the bag but Topping, the dour, dogged policeman, required some solid, definite proof to substantiate what they had told him. He was sure he was on the right track, close to at least one body, and was understandably annoyed at what he saw as the unwarranted rantings of an uninformed Press that was slowly turning against him.

With impeccable timing, on the afternoon of Wednesday, 1 July 1987, in a week that the *Manchester Evening News* had dismissed the whole affair as a 'farce', he got his result.

Topping was once more interviewing Brady at Ashworth when the spadework of his carefully chosen squad unearthed a white stiletto shoe in the peat of Hollin Brow Knoll, close to the border between Lancashire and Yorkshire. He was informed by mobile phone and took great delight in telling the man he was interrogating that there had been a major development. There can be little doubt that this was the most important moment in his professional life and he was going to enjoy his vindication.

I got a call at the hospital that they'd found a body and was advised to make my way up after six p.m. when the scrum of reporters hanging about would have gone away. They were told that nothing significant had happened and the diggers got into their police cars and drove off, secretly leaving just one man behind to guard the site. The last thing Topping wanted was a media circus when his inquiry was at such a crucial stage. When I arrived, two reporters who had obviously been tipped off were waiting but I took them for police officers and asked where I should be heading. They said: 'Over in that direction,' pointing across a hill, and seemed quite calm about it all. I wasn't.

The grave was 250 yards from the main cross-Pennine route above Saddleworth. It was a clear evening, as it had been twenty-four years previously, almost to the day.

Up there the ground undulates gently, rising and falling, with mile after mile of grassy fields rolling like a green sea. In early summer it can be attractive, but it never loses that eerie, bleak aura that conjures an inescapable feeling of dread. Not many people go to the moor at night. If the Moors Murderers had wanted to create a dramatic, menacing effect they chose their graveyard well.

The road from Saddleworth winds slowly upwards, with large, old trees leaning over on either side. At first it is rather friendly and charming, with shafts of sunlight sparkling through the branches, the light flickering like a strobe as you drive. Then, with greater altitude, the woods slowly give way to the sparser moorland and, in the last mile or so before the top, there are no trees to block the panoramic view as the land dips towards farms before rising to a distant curve.

The rough grass that stretches endlessly on either side of the road is marked with the tops of massive granite rocks that look as though they are striving to release themselves, to force their way to the surface. Enormous mounds of solid stone, all a deep, depressing grey, buried for millennia, captives of the moor.

At the top, where the police cars were, I had to put on my heavy boots before marching out towards the cluster of men hidden from me on the other side of the rise. It was, I remember, a nice evening for a stroll.

Up a hill, watching my step, moving carefully across a flat piece of ground, I could feel the peat shifting underfoot, shuddering each time I placed a boot down. It was like walking on the chest of a fat man breathing gently as he slept. I couldn't help but wonder how on earth the police had managed to find anything in this desolate expanse.

Pauline was still buried, lying in a small hollow, one foot and shoe protruding for all the world like a marker. All we could see was the shoe but none of us had the slightest doubt what lay before us here. Each man on the hill knew what this young girl used to look like and what clothes she had been wearing the last time she had kissed her mother goodbye. We knew what she used to be, all those years ago. The question was: What was left?

From a forensic point of view she was in remarkable shape. She had spent a quarter of a century a few inches below the surface of a patch of land that was snowbound in winter, parched in summer, soaking in spring and wind-blown in autumn. Above ground this is among the harshest landscapes in Britain. Yet below, ironically, she had been protected by the peat that kept out the weather, the heat, the cold, the scavenging animals and, most importantly, the bacteria.

The microbes only got the opportunity to begin their work when we got Pauline out of her makeshift tomb.

It didn't take long to clear the earth from around the body and we could see many things straight away. Not least was that this was indeed Pauline Reade. Her mother, her father, and her brother, Paul, could all quite easily have identified her if it had been necessary. I noticed later, when I saw Paul at the inquest, that there was a distinct family resemblance.

The family members would have also noticed immediately, had they seen her, that her throat had been cut.

Fortunately, they were spared the need to view what Pauline had become. They would always remember the vivacious teenager with the broad, easy grin, full of life, and not this sad, pitiful sight, tanned dark, a three-dimensional shadow of what she had once been.

Usually at a death, the only feelings I allow myself are the unavoidable sadness and, just occasionally, a sense of revulsion. This time, though, I felt a surge of excitement as I realized we were about to try to resolve a secret that was of massive public interest.

As the excavation continued and the peat was gently peeled aside, Pauline was revealed lying on her left side, facing the main road. Her head was slightly retracted and her left arm was folded across the front of her body with her hand on her right shoulder. Her right arm lay along her side.

The thighs were extended and the knees were bent so that Pauline's heels were tucked up close to her buttocks. The right shoe, the one that had led to the discovery, was in place but the other was resting on her thigh, clearly positioned there by the hand of her murderer before she was covered over with earth.

Pauline was wearing a heavy woollen coat. The skirt and underslip were pulled up above her waist and we could see stockings with suspenders at mid-thigh but no knickers or suspender belt. She had been wearing a suspender belt the night she had vanished.

As the body was moved gingerly on to a plastic sheet to wrap it up and take it to Oldham mortuary, the right hand, the wrist joint ruined by time, became detached. It was a sharp reminder that this might be a complex task.

An hour later, with the body safely under lock and key, we went home and prepared for the following day.

It had been agreed that, should a find be made, the post-mortem would be carried out by both myself, as the pathologist for the area, and Dr (now Professor) Mike Green, from Leeds University. He had worked with the original Moors inquiry pathology team, Professor Cyril John Polson and Dr David Gee.

In a bizarre coincidence, the day after they had finished their examination of John Kilbride at Saddleworth mortuary in 1965, a heavy snowfall prevented the pathologist for the Huddersfield area getting to work. As the road was passable from the Manchester side, I was asked to cover for one of his jobs and travelled up to Saddleworth to confirm a heart-attack case.

When I finished, the mortician wrote down in the ledger the date, 22 October, the name of the patient, the cause of death, and my own name. Immediately above it were the names of the other two Moors victims, Lesley Ann Downey's examination dated 16 October and John Kilbride's dated 21 October.

Instead of describing their causes of death the mortician had written the stark single word 'Murder' in the ledger. It was clear that both children had died from violent means but the extensive decomposition of the bodies precluded the post-mortems from establishing the precise cause of death.

I had never imagined that I would get any closer to the case than that juxtaposition of names. But at 1.45 p.m. on Thursday, 2 July 1987, Mike Green and I began the task of trying to work out how Pauline had come to lie dead with Lesley Ann and John.

Bits of peat and soil that had stuck to the clothing were brushed away and the coat was carefully cut off with scissors. All the clothes were given to forensic expert Dr Karen Mashiter who did a remarkably good job of reconstructing the items and proving that they had belonged to Pauline.

The removal of the coat revealed a handknitted cardigan that was also cut away, but we left the sleeves in place. They would act like a false skin to hold the tissue and bone structure of the arms together. The left hand became detached now and it was clear that although the body was in relatively remarkable shape there had been, as expected, major deterioration.

Under the cardigan were a black blouse and lurex patterned skirt. A brassiere was fastened at the back, and a slip and nylon net petticoat were intact. The skin was tanned to the consistency of leather and began to crack at the joints of the knees, at the waist and the neck – essentially wherever the body bent. All this restricted the examination.

Underneath the collar of the cardigan was a small section of gold chain, broken off from the rest of its length. There was a deep cut across the front of the throat and the coat collar, with its lining, had been pushed into the wound. Whatever force had done that had taken with it the rest of the chain, which we found inside.

This was our initial investigation. But it was clear that the body was going to deteriorate further and decompose rapidly now that it was in the open air.

Dr Green had made a number of inquiries among people who had worked on retrieved long-buried bodies. Only two years previously the 2,000-year-old body of a man had been uncovered in Wilmslow, Cheshire, and the experiences of the archaeologists and other scientists who had dealt with it proved very useful.

Advice was also gleaned from experts who had worked on the project to raise Henry VIII's flagship, the *Mary Rose*. The warship sank off Portsmouth in the sixteenth century and lay buried and preserved in mud for 447 years. When raised in 1982 a way of preserving its timbers with a chemical similar to antifreeze had been found.

It was vital to prevent the body's skin drying and cracking so it was placed in a brown metal casket containing a softening fluid similar to that used on the wood, polyethylene glycol PEG 600 with added water and bicarbonate at pH8, slightly alkaline to reduce the natural acidity of the peat. A friend of Topping's worked as head of security at Shell Chemicals at nearby Carrington and they kindly supplied a variation on antifreeze. Before we could do any more the body had to stay immersed, floating in the solution, for nearly a week.

Every day outside the mortuary I was greeted by a posse of reporters, all wanting to know what was happening. I told them, truthfully, that absolutely nothing was happening, but I suspect a few didn't believe me.

On Wednesday, 8 July, we took the body out and placed it on the metal table once more. It was now possible to extend the legs and arms and realign the head and neck.

Only the lower legs and knees had not been immersed and these were still hard but there was nothing of significance for us to look at there.

Laid out straight for the first time, the body's height was measured at a little under five feet five inches. It was clear now there were two parallel knife wounds to the neck, one very severe, three inches below the point of the chin, and a second, less deep, two inches below that. In addition there was a swelling on the forehead the diameter of a kitchen mug. Pauline had been hit hard on the head.

Internal examination showed that one of the throat cuts had been delivered with such force that it severed the spinal cord. The angle of the cuts, horizontal rather than angled upwards to one side or another, suggested that they were not self-inflicted and had been carried out by another individual. Evidentially, this was important.

The facial bones showed all the elements you would expect in a teenager. As people get older these bones knit together at a fairly specific rate. They showed that this was a girl of approximately Pauline's age. That was hardly a surprise but it was another piece of recorded evidence to help the coroner, Bryan North, come to his conclusions. The teeth and jaw also confirmed her age.

There was no other sign of injury we could detect and, such was the extent of the body's deterioration, we were not able to investigate whether there had been any sexual assault.

At the inquest our conclusions were stated as follows: 'We are satisfied that this is the body of Pauline Reade. Although no positive medical or dental identification can be made, the clothing and personal possessions have been positively identified. The X-rays of the bones show epiphysial union consistent with an age of approximately sixteen years. Direct inspection of the sutures of the skull tends to support this estimate of age.

'The appearance of the neck is consistent with homicidal cut throat. There are two separate incised wounds running horizontally across the midline, one four inches in length which gapes and one more superficial, two inches in length. There are no tentative incisions. They do not run upwards towards either ear and on the left side the upper incised wound almost completely divides the stemomastoid muscle and appears to involve the anterior surface of the cervical spine.

'The swelling in the centre of the forehead appears to be a haematoma and is consistent with the application of blunt force, either with a fist or an instrument. There is no mark upon the skin to give any further assistance.

'Post-mortem deterioration of the perineum and anus precludes any examination for sexual assault.

'The general state of the preservation of the body is consistent with immersion in an acid peat bog for twenty to thirty years.

'The pushing of the collar of the coat into the wound of the neck appears to have been deliberate rather than accidental during the burial of the body and could well have been carried out in an attempt to reduce the amount of bleeding.'

Topping was pleased with our findings. They confirmed for him that what he had gleaned from Hindley and Brady about Pauline's fate was basically the truth. Ironically, his finest hour was followed quickly by his leaving the police force. His efforts digging on the moor had exacerbated an old back injury and he retired almost immediately on the grounds of ill health.

In the hours that Dr Green and I had been working on Pauline's body, it was physically changing, degenerating, liquefying under our gaze as nature at last began to take its proper course.

For twenty-four years so little had happened to Pauline as she lay in darkness, but now she was in the light, delivered from that confining grave. Now her truth was finally told and it seemed, somehow, that, as her body began its inevitable, overdue return to dust, her captured spirit was simultaneously set free.

2

A Savage Breeze

On a bright August morning a summer breeze fanned the flames of disaster and claimed the lives of fifty-five people in less than the time it would take to recite their names.

Shortly before seven o'clock on that terrible day in 1985, six crew members and 131 passengers boarded a Corfu-bound holiday jet at Manchester Airport.

The tourists, laden with duty-free purchases, some already in their shorts and T-shirts, a few boisterous, all excited, were looking forward to the best part of their year. The vast majority had got up in the middle of the night to get to Ringway for a five a.m. check-in, but the holiday adrenalin, mixed with the natural apprehension everyone has about flying, soon dispelled any cobwebs.

More than a couple of trippers would have taken advantage of the early-opening bar in the international departure lounge to have a snifter to steady their nerves. Although statistics show you are much more likely to be hit by lightning than to die in a plane crash, a lot of people have a fear of flying.

For a few of those on board it was going to be their first flight, for others their longest. Corfu was four hours away, a long time in the air, twice as far as the Spanish Costas. The stewardesses went through the routine of explaining emergency procedures and what to do in the unlikely event of an accident, and then spent time, as usual, reassuring those few who looked a little green around the gills.

Finally, with everything stowed properly in the overhead lockers or under the seats, with all the seat backs upright and with everyone securely strapped in, flight KT 328 began its doomed journey, pushing back off the stand and taxiing smoothly towards Runway 24. The plane was virtually full, with passengers seated across the fuselage in rows of six seats divided by a narrow aisle, three seats to each side. Like all holiday charters it felt a bit like being in a sardine tin.

Captain Peter Terrington, a vastly experienced former RAF flyer, had piloted the British Airtours Boeing 737 to Barcelona the previous day and had noticed that the number one engine had a low idling speed. But everything checked out, everything was by the book, the engineers were happy and there was no reason to suspect a serious fault. The pre-flight checks indicated that the aircraft was ready for take-off.

What Captain Terrington couldn't know was that, deep within the powerful Pratt and Whitney JT8D-IS engine, a weakness had developed, a fatal weakness. A crack around its circumference was not going to be able to withstand the awesome heat and pressure about to be created by the jet systems as they produced sufficient power to defy gravity and hurl the aircraft skyward. A catastrophe was inevitable.

The plane, with its name, *River Orin*, printed proudly high up near the cockpit, turned at the head of the runway. As the pilot brought the nose around, passengers could see the landing lights stretching before them along the two-mile-long strip.

With the turn completed, Captain Terrington thrust the

throttles forward. The pitch of the engine noise rose, the whole aircraft, code name Juliet Lima, rumbled and shifted as power grew, and then, at 7.12 a.m. British Summer Time, the brakes were released and it hurtled forward, accelerating like a racing car.

Some passengers closed their eyes, some continued to read their papers, most looked out of the windows, saw the airport terminal rushing past and thought of Greek islands, sunshine and two weeks off work. Everyone would have been waiting for that critical moment when the long tube of the fuselage tilted and the wheels left the ground. It was a moment that never came.

As the *River Orin* touched 144 m.p.h., thirty-two seconds after it had started its run, there was a loud bang that all the crew immediately thought was a bursting tyre.

Reacting instantly, the captain decided to abort take-off and informed the air traffic controllers that he was stopping. Airport staff in the tower who looked out at this point saw what Captain Terrington could not: that there was a fire in or near the engine under the left wing.

To stop as quickly as possible the captain closed down both throttles and selected reverse thrust. Still concerned about tyres, he warned the first officer to be careful as he slammed on the footbrake.

From the main concourse horrified onlookers could see a large plume of grey-black smoke trailing behind the aircraft. On board, the cockpit fire-warning bell sounded. At this stage only forty-five seconds had elapsed since take-off had begun.

Within the affected engine, one of the nine two-feet-long combustion chambers had split asunder, rupturing its outer casing and, crucially, sending pieces of metal shrapnel shooting upwards to punch an eight-inch hole in a fuel-tank access panel in the wing. High-octane kerosene poured out, igniting in the superheated air and, even before the aircraft stopped, the white-hot jet flame began to burn through the side of the plane.

Passengers at the front didn't realize the scale of the problem for several moments. But those on the left and especially at the back quickly realized they were in real mortal danger. It was at the rear where the vast majority died.

Of the twenty-three people sitting furthest back in rows 19, 20, 21 and 22, the only two to survive were seated in 19B and 20B. Both told investigators they unclipped their safety belts before the plane had come to a halt and started to move forward very early in the emergency.

Of a total of forty-three people sitting in rows 16 to 22, that is, from six rows behind the overwing exit to the back of the fuselage, only six escaped. Thirteen more died in the six rows ahead of them and the last five fatalities were in rows 7, 8 and 9. Everyone in the first six rows lived. Clearly, seat position was a crucial factor in deciding whether a passenger was a victim or a survivor.

At 7.14 a.m., as soon as the aircraft came to rest, the purser tried to open the front right-hand exit but it jammed, caught in the cover of the inflatable slide. He went straight to the left-hand exit, opened that successfully and then returned to sort out the other door. The delay was only between ten and twenty seconds. But, in the context of the speed of events, that was a significant period of time, worsening the problem of frightened passengers bunching together, their cramped environment slowing their progress out of the plane.

The moment the pilot halted on a slipway just off the runway, several windows that had already begun to honeycomb and melt surrendered to the intense heat. Flames entered the narrow, crowded passenger cabin with what was described by those there as a 'blowtorch' effect. Panic was total, terror absolute. There could have been no other emotions.

The rear door on the right, the side away from the fire, opened a second or two before the *River Orin* stopped, but the wind prevented anyone using it. It was only the slightest breeze, entirely inconsequential to the aircraft normally, but it was blowing the fire from the wing towards the fuselage, diagonally towards the back of the plane. As the door opened, flames were already enveloping the whole of the back section and were now channelled in through the opening.

The heat was so intense, the destruction so rapid, that within seventy seconds of flight KT 328 coming to a halt the plane's rear section disintegrated and crumbled to the ground.

Within seconds, nine people died, purely from the lethal effects of the searing heat. The temperature rose so quickly in their section of the aircraft that their circulation systems ceased to function. Each had some evidence in their bodies of the toxic fumes that filled the cabin, but the amount they had inhaled was insufficient to be fatal. They didn't live long enough to take that many breaths.

Toxicology tests carried out by RAF scientists showed that twenty more died from the combined effects of the fire and the fumes, but only twenty-six of the victims were killed by the poisonous effects of the gases alone.

Undoubtedly, everyone who died in this disaster became

unconscious extremely quickly and all bar three were dead one or two minutes later. One person showed signs of life for five minutes, a second for thirty-four minutes and a third, apparently a very fit man, died in hospital six days later.

Before take-off, the plane had been topped up with nearly 4,000 gallons of fuel, stored in tanks in the wings and fuselage. Within thirty seconds of it stopping on the slipway, firefighters were pouring foam onto the blazing engine and the flames initially died down. But the fuel continued to stream out of the wing. As it splashed onto the hot engine, it once again exploded into a destructive blaze.

At first, passengers in the front seats, up ahead of the fire, had little idea of what was happening behind them. But at the back there was pandemonium.

There were three viable exits, the two at the front and one over the right-hand wing. Both rear exits were useless, as was the one over the left wing. Everyone was pushing to get forward – and then the smoke came in like a shroud and no one could see where 'forward' was.

A solid snake of dense, black, hot smoke ran rapidly along the roof of the cabin above everyone's heads, hit the forward bulkhead, curled over and started coming back like a demonic fist.

Seats burst into flames, walls melted and overhead racks dripped fire. Carbon monoxide and hydrogen cyanide polluted what was left of the air, their suffocating effects confusing and debilitating, driving the will to run, to escape, to survive from passengers' screaming minds. Some people sat down in this version of Hell, craving sleep.

Much of the internal fabric reduced in moments to tiny airborne particles that floated like a million hot insects, solidifying on contact with skin, turning gluey, clogging eyes and ears, gagging throats, collecting in mouths with the consistency of Oxo cubes.

Some people would have held their breath if only they had known what was coming. But the foul vapour engulfed them too fast and, with nothing in their lungs, they had no choice but to inhale the vile, poisoned atmosphere. With each reluctant breath another victim fell and, among the fallen, only a precious few ever saw light again.

All but two of the survivors were evacuated by 7.18 a.m., six minutes after the aircraft had begun take-off. By this time, on any other day, the passengers would have still been looking at a glowing 'fasten seat belt' sign and listening to the clatter in the galley as stewardesses prepared to serve a hot breakfast out of silver foil trays.

Firemen pulled another survivor out ninety seconds later. Fifteen minutes after that, when it was believed everyone left on board was dead, the last survivor was discovered under a pile of bodies, his chest heaving as he struggled to breathe.

Up to then the firemen had been following procedures that would help the crash investigators, noting the position of each body so that the distances they travelled from their seats to the point where they fell could be plotted. It was not much, but every small piece of information could assist in the development of further safety improvements.

When they discovered the man who was still alive twenty-two and a half minutes after the aborted take-off all that changed and they simply got all the bodies out as swiftly as possible. No others had survived. The man they had found, the last survivor of flight KT 328, was the one to finally lose his struggle for life six days later in hospital.

I heard about the disaster on the news and waited for the call to go to the airport.

Inquiries were made about using the Manchester mortuary for the autopsies. Although it could have coped with the numbers, it would have meant that all other work would have been brought to a halt. In the end, it was decided to use a hangar close to the site of the accident, one normally used to store snowploughs.

A team of RAF pathologists was called in because of their experience with air crashes. But, because this plane had never actually left the ground, the deaths became a matter for the Manchester coroner, Leonard Gorodkin, and myself as the Home Office pathologist for the area.

As my colleague, Dr Bill Lawler, was on holiday, two experienced pathologists from local hospitals, Professor John McLure from Withington Hospital and Dr Dan De Kretser from North Manchester General were drafted in. We gathered at the airport police station to decide how best to carry out our two tasks of establishing causes of death and assisting where necessary with identifying bodies.

It was agreed dentists would go in first, charting fillings. But as we had a good idea who everyone was from the passenger list a relatively simple cursory dental examination was sufficient.

There were to be three pathology teams, working simultaneously. Each consisted of two senior policemen, one to take notes and the second to collect belongings and valuables, a police photographer to record the injuries, a civilian pathologist and an RAF pathologist.

The makeshift mortuary was a distance from the main concourse, to the right of the runway. I remember driving there behind a police escort in my 3-series BMW.

The airport: always busy, always noisy with businessmen, holidaymakers, hundreds of staff, security men, baggage handlers, people rushing and eating and chatting and calling to one another and chasing their children, shopping, waiting, reading, ringing home. The airport: constantly buzzing with the background noise of take-off and landing, taxiing, revving cars, lights, people, life.

Now the airport was dead.

Not a sound, not a person, not a car, nothing moving. I can't remember a more complete quiet. Manchester Airport's huge complex sits within a few hundred yards of a motorway, there are houses at the end of the runway, it is on the edge of the biggest housing estate in Europe. Even when shut down there should have been background noise, things intruding from outside. But on this day of mourning it was cloaked in an all-pervading silence: absolute quiet, noiseless as thought.

The hangar loomed ahead, its size peculiarly threatening and growing bigger as we neared the vast doors. To one side the burned, blackened hulk of the aircraft was starkly alone, a dreadful and pitiful sight, lying like a broken animal half picked clean by scavengers.

None of us wanted to walk into that hangar. It was a strange feeling, a fear certainly, but of what, I didn't know. Beyond the door was the stuff of my daily routine, the bodies of the dead that required clinical observation. Yet somehow this seemed different.

But it was more than just the numbers that made the difference. That any single individual should die has its own sadness and significance. That fifty-five should die in a day for their own unrelated reasons is no less or more tragic.

But that fifty-five should perish at the same time, in the same horrific manner, in seconds, together, almost as one entity, because nature, timing, human frailty and chance conspired to produce a disaster multiplied the feeling of loss beyond all usual boundaries. I was overwhelmed with a deep sense of sorrow.

The door rolled back. Oddly, in the vastness of the cold, metal building the plastic-sheeted bodies on stretchers on the floor didn't seem to take up that much space. Each of us breathed heavily once or twice but we all knew that the only way forward was to be totally professional, totally clinical.

We had three trestle tables set up in a line. The civilian and RAF pathologists in each team took it in turns to carry out the physically arduous task of dissection. The RAF technicians did an excellent job of keeping us supplied with new, sharp instruments. After the third or fourth body, scalpels go blunt.

We had agreed that it was best to try to do the whole job in one go, minimizing any delay in releasing the bodies to their relatives. The funerals could be held and the families' time for grieving could begin. The quicker it began, the sooner the pain would start to ebb.

We started at 3.30 p.m.

By midnight, exhausted, we had finished and were relieved that it was over. None of us would have relished going home only to have to return for more of the same the following day. We could now escape.

The tragedy was so enormous that it somehow had a presence, a genuine substance that touched us all with a clammy finger. Each noise in the hangar echoed from ground to roof and back, the piercing cry of angry souls clamouring in the eaves like whirling birds, demanding answers, accusing everyone, forgiving no one.

For the one and only time in my career I had felt almost nervous among the dead, sensitive to their former being. Their lives were clearly gone, but the questions over their deaths lingered in the atmosphere in an unnervingly, almost tangible fashion.

As expected, the examinations were relatively straightforward from the point of view of deciding the cause of death. The victims had died because of the fire.

What was important, however, was that we established no one had suffered injuries other than those caused by the blaze, no one had broken an arm or leg in the mêlée and become incapacitated in a way not directly involving the fire. Also no one had died of a heart attack or any other natural cause.

We were eventually able to show the crash investigators that everyone who had died on the flight had been prevented from getting off alive purely by the effects of the smoke, fumes and flames. That was an important factor in the consequent attempts to improve aircraft safety in the wake of the Manchester disaster.

The success, from a technical point of view, of the makeshift mortuary led to a decision to keep bodies at the airport in the – hopefully unlikely – event of another disaster occurring. Now, however, drains and guttering have been built into the buildings to improve medical working conditions and adaptable tables of an appropriate design for autopsies have been made available.

A 'dummy run' was organized as a practice for the unthinkable, with police, fire, ambulance, hospitals and every other possible service that could be involved. Based on the premise that two aircraft had collided at the end of the runway this rehearsal quickly became something of a fiasco.

Volunteers who acted out the parts of the victims had the extent of their injury written on a note that was stuck to their foreheads with sticky tape. Logically enough, those marked 'dead' were left alone so that the rescuers could concentrate on the living. Unfortunately, since the 'dead' were still breathing and were left lying out in the open, immobile on cold grass during an unseasonably cool evening, a number of them began to develop the early stages of hypothermia.

Eventually the paramedics attending the dummy crash had to abandon their make-believe victims and turn their attentions to the scores of shivering individuals with 'dead' stickers plastered to their heads. Luckily, with so many medics around, everyone got the very best treatment.

In his report on the genuine disaster, Wing Commander Ian Hill, from the Air Force pathology team, insisted that it was a totally survivable accident. He concluded that, given an identical wing explosion, it should be possible to get everyone off a Boeing 737 alive.

The burning fabric had produced carbon monoxide and hydrogen cyanide gases, both of which proved fatal to some passengers, but at lower levels the effects of the fumes had also caused incapacitation, preventing people from getting out. Since the disaster, much work has been carried out on developing alternative materials for aircraft furniture and fittings.

Escape routes were inadequate and, according to Hill, were 'directly responsible for the loss of life'. Again, there have been improvements in access to aircraft exits, with better lighting for passengers to follow routes to safety and more space in the exit approaches. Pilots also have instructions to bear in mind the wind direction in cases of fire. The official report into the accident, published three and a half years after the deaths, listed thirty-one separate safety improvements, most of which were accepted without question by the Civil Aviation Authority. However, at the time of writing, several years on, many arguments still rage about what else should be done to make flying safer still.

Today, not least because of what was learned at Manchester, air travel is safer than ever before and, despite what I saw, I am not afraid of flying.

But I must admit I'm always glad when, having collected my hand luggage, I get to the top of the steps and someone in a smart suit smiles and says: 'Thanks for flying with us, sir. We look forward to seeing you again.'

3

Mother Mac's

The most ordinary people are sometimes driven to commit the most extraordinary acts of violence.

Until that final, devastating step they appear perfectly normal, average, unremarkable. They are 'the neighbours', or the 'friends from down the road', or 'that couple, you know, what's-his-name'.

He could be the chap you've been drinking with in the local, the one who rarely overdoes it, the one who just occasionally flies off the handle but is basically harmless.

Or he might be that bloke in the football team who always cracks the bad jokes in the changing rooms and manages to keep a manic grin on his face even when his team's been thrashed 4–0. Then there's the guy, you remember the one, who's always washing his car and keeps his lawn perfect. His kids are always so well turned out and his wife is that quiet, mousy woman who could be so pretty if she'd only make an effort, but he doesn't seem to mind as he obviously dotes on her.

Or, in your nightmares, he lives in your house, and you can't believe your eyes. You recoil at your knowledge.

'Someone out there knows this man.' So often the news broadcasts are filled with this phrase as police appeal desperately for information. 'He may be heavily bloodstained . . . if you at all suspect . . . please come forward . . . in complete confidence . . . I appeal to anyone who thinks . . . he could strike again . . .'

Every killer who ever drew breath lived alongside people who thought they knew him, understood him, people who were his friends, his relatives, his father, mother, wife, children. Those he leaves alive are shocked, disbelieving and devastated. In the beginning murderers are invariably ordinary people: babies are not born to kill.

When a detective is faced with a suspicious death, the people he turns to first are the immediate members of the family. This is not because he's offering help and counselling. It's because they are his initial prime suspects.

Murders are usually committed for one of three main reasons: pleasure, an evil delight in taking the life of another, often involving a perverse sexual motive; greed, the need to get rid of someone to take what is in their possession, be it goods, position or another person; and passion, an eruption of emotion caused by any number of stimuli. Of the three, the last motivates by far the greatest number of slayings.

Of 'passionate' killings, the majority are domestic, not least because it is considerably easier to get annoyed with someone close to you than with someone you've just met. And sometimes, when the anger finally surfaces, it does so with a ferocity few of us can begin to comprehend.

A man can inflict the most dreadful damage on those who for so long have been closest to him: his parents, brother, sister, wife and, sadly, much too often, his children.

Every case is different, obviously, but there are a number of identifiable threads that run through most such killings. Usually the victim isn't directly responsible for his or her fate.

Although the act of violence may be the culmination of an argument, the true reasons for the explosion of savagery usually run much deeper and are self-propagated rather than reactive. Monsters have a lengthy gestation period.

The assailant is typically almost always close to rock bottom in self-esteem, a loser, professionally and personally, and often trapped in a downward emotional spiral that crushes what little humanity he has left, dragging him ever lower, ever deeper into depression. He may in fact be no better or worse off materially than most of us but a crucial factor is his implacable belief in his own failure. Reality can seem like a subjective thing: your own 'truth' is the only one that counts.

From these depths of self-loathing and despair grow cruel spiritual tentacles. Each in turn chokes a portion of what had previously made up a normal, everyday personality and sets in its place a fearsome readiness to commit an act of vengeance, to rail against the unfairness of it all – to strike out.

In most cases the lethal assault comes suddenly, like an ugly jack-in-the-box springing out when the emotional trigger is finally pulled by any small thing: a chance remark, a casual rebuke. A simple glance can be enough to release wild, unstoppable fury. The deterioration from unremarkable neighbour to foul murderer may take years but rarely reveals itself publicly until the final, dreadful moment of truth.

The immediate family, often doomed to be the victims, might notice apparently minor differences in the behaviour of Dad, or Cousin George or Uncle Bob. But people on the outside see the same old guy, telling his jokes, buying his round, being himself – until he strikes.

The psychologists tell us that in many cases the killer is, with a perverse logic, attacking *himself* with each blow he brings down on his victim. But, since he remains physically uninjured, there is nothing to stop him continuing the assault. You hear of 'frenzied attacks' when people were stabbed numerous times, when the third or fourth wound was fatal but the attacker kept going, his eyes closed, hacking and slicing blindly until he himself collapsed, exhausted by the effort, or the blade of his weapon snapped.

More often than not, his violence spent, the killer will insist that he can remember nothing at all of the event. He will claim to have no knowledge of the actual bestial savagery: several minutes or even longer periods of time are, he says, completely blank.

Without doubt, this is sometimes a cynical defence ploy. But often the amnesia will be genuine. There are many reasons for wanting to block out such a memory: entire essays have been written on the multi-layered methods by which the human mind defends itself, refusing to accept information that might prove unbearable. Without delving into the complexities of these mental acrobatics it can hardly be surprising that some mentally disturbed killers find a psychological escape route when they finally open their eyes to see the appalling results of their activities.

Having been confronted too often by the horrific consequences of such behaviour, it comes as no surprise whatsoever to me that any mind with even the tiniest vestige of sanity left would look for a way to block out the image of what it has done, to try to deny an undoubted moment of evil.

People often ask how I cope with what they consider to be the gory side of my work. But I must freely admit that it is really only in the rarest circumstances that the state of a dead person upsets me on a personal level. There have been a few, some of which you will read about in this volume, but in most cases it is relatively simple to keep things clinical.

All I get, no matter what it looks like, is the end result of the whole affair. The carnage is usually very hard on the eye, certainly. But I'm spared the pain, the anguish, the heartache and the suffering. All that has gone before.

I believe it is more disturbing to have to work directly with the terminally ill than to deal with a person for whom pain and fear are things of the past. The living suffer more than the dead. I did see some patients who came in for tests in the normal way of hospital life but, usually, the closest I got to emotional pain was with the relatives of the dead.

Occasionally they came to me for a reason, for some solid information to store with the rest of their memories. As part of the process of grieving they wanted to know, needed to know, to *understand* what it was that had claimed this life they had treasured. In simple language, what had been the cause of death. A colleague once described my profession as 'physician to the bereaved'. It is an apt phrase.

Like thousands of medical practitioners I am trained to take a scalpel and open people up. I spend much of my day cutting into human bodies, removing and examining samples of tissue from hearts, lungs, kidneys and livers. I check the ingredients of a victim's last meal. I weigh brains.

Consequently, to me the sight of blood and sliced organs is neither rare nor shocking. If doctors fainted at the sight of blood we'd be in serious trouble. I got into pathology, the study of tissue, because I considered that it was the purest form of medicine. My job at Oldham General Hospital was to get right to the heart of the disease, the infection, the problem. I concerned myself with the microscopic reality of what was happening to a body and tried to locate the cause of the illness rather than becoming preoccupied with its symptoms, its effects upon the patient.

Equally with murder cases, the work I do takes into account nothing connected with the lifestyle of the individual. I am left only to ponder, once I have my results, how that lifestyle might have contributed to bringing about what had happened to this or that body. Each disfiguring mark, while far from attractive, provides a piece of information that I regard, not with distaste, but with professional interest. There is no point in recoiling from a corpse. The dead can't hurt you.

Actually, without exception, the shocking part is never the body itself. What shocks me is the thought of the terrible rage that can make one human being do such things to another, particularly to one they professed to love.

In the cold winter of 1969, shortly after I had become Home Office pathologist, I was called to a terraced house in Sixth Street, Trafford Park. This is a dull, disappointing residential area built to service a giant industrial estate, once the biggest in Europe, developed around the success of the Manchester Ship Canal but now faded, in decline.

As always at crime scenes, there were policemen all over the place. One officer guarding the front door politely allowed me past him into the grey living room.

At murders one can often detect a casual 'been there, seen that' attitude among the officers. This is partly, no doubt, because they like to project a macho image. But also, I suspect, it helps them get through the difficulties that most people have when dealing with death.

Here, however, there were no smart remarks, no casual one-liners or tasteless gags, not a smile, not a wink, not a single friendly wave or pat on the back. In this house everyone was strictly business.

There was blood on the front door, on the porch and on the door leading from the lounge to the kitchen. A pane of clear glass in the door panel had cracked. In the kitchen was an empty pan with potatoes, ready for cooking, to one side. A meat cleaver, heavily bloodstained, lay untouched by the detectives.

The doorway, its door open, led to a typically small yard, stone-flagged, walled on each side, with a wooden gate straight ahead of me that would open onto the back alleyway. On the ground was the body of a boy aged just fifteen months.

The toddler, clothed in a bib, blue overalls, a blue cardigan and a towelling nappy, lay with his head pointing towards the door, towards me. The child looked ludicrously small to have suffered such terrible damage. It was almost as if there was more injury than infant.

He had wounds to the left side of his head, exposing the bone and revealing obvious fractures. His left ear had been effectively severed. A metal coal chisel, half an inch in diameter, was protruding from the front of his neck and sticking out the other side, two inches below the child's left ear, like an embedded missile.

Surprisingly, the chisel, though it looked devastating, had caused almost no serious damage, missing major veins, arteries and the spinal column. If that had been the youngster's only injury he would almost certainly have lived.

The damage had already been done by the meat cleaver.

The father, who meekly gave himself up, had just been told that he would have to go into hospital as a psychiatric patient. His awful response to that news showed clearly that the diagnosis of paranoid schizophrenia was correct, though, tragically, far too late.

Another terrifying passion built up in the mind of a Manchester pub landlord who was already inclined towards violence but, nevertheless, was regarded warmly by his mates as 'one of the lads'. Neighbours recalled that when Arthur Bradbury and his family lived in Leyland Street, Harpurhey, they were 'nice people', a 'happy family'. When they all moved into Mother Mac's pub in the centre of the city there was no reason for that view to alter.

Arthur, just thirty when he died, was remembered by regulars as a quietly spoken man, calm and sensible but one who could be very outspoken on certain issues. He liked a half of mild but was not a heavy drinker.

The pub, his first and only, had in years past been called The Wellington. But its name had been changed in 1969 in honour of a former landlady, a popular Manchester character, 'Mother' Mac McLennon, who, after the death of her husband, took the place on and made it an institution. Eventually she had to retire and Arthur took over the tenancy in 1985, moving into the upstairs living accommodation with his wife, Maureen, their six-year-old daughter, Alison, and Maureen's two sons from a previous marriage, Andrew and James, aged thirteen and eleven.

Arthur had earlier unsuccessfully attempted to run a boarding house on the Isle of Man, so he was delighted when Whitbread installed him in what was a rough but successful pub.

At first everything seemed to go well. The former regular soldier chucked out a few troublemakers, barred a number of difficult drunks and brought a level of respectability back to the establishment.

Profits, however, did not keep up with previous performance and the men from the brewery were soon suspicious. Only eight months into the business, Arthur received his first serious warning from his bosses. His stocks were down and he was informed in no uncertain terms what standards were required.

Briefly, things improved. But then they deteriorated just as quickly and in the middle of May, shortly before his thirtieth birthday, Arthur was told he was to be fired. He was put on two months' notice and informed he had to be out by 19 July.

It was only one more pressure among many. Perhaps his army experiences had left him damaged, maybe something from his childhood sparked it all off. We'll never know, but it is fair to suspect that this event, although his own fault, injured him, and the self-inflicted wound festered at a rapid rate, his hatred mixing with his anger and frustration to melt hotly into a congealed, dangerous, venomous thing.

The man's tendency towards violence, police later discovered, was most obvious in his attitude towards his wife. Maureen's hairdresser told detectives that Maureen had confessed to her that Arthur had attempted to strangle her with a telephone wire. More than one person told of seeing the landlady in the pub with the occasional black eye or red weal on her neck. Too often, her make-up had been applied heavily to conceal yet another bruise. With typical working-class pride she would try to hide the damage from strangers. But she was sufficiently angry with her husband's behaviour to complain to her friends.

During the same period, staff at Mother Mac's described how one day they found the living quarters half wrecked after Arthur had thrown chairs around in a tantrum, turning over tables and smashing the telephone into little pieces, enraged over nothing more than a cracked fish bowl.

When things had gone wrong for him before, at the Isle of Man boarding house, his response on returning to Manchester had been to set fire to clothes and furniture in an attempt to burn his house down, possibly hoping for an insurance pay-out. He had failed on that occasion but a pattern was developing. Arthur Bradbury, friend to many, cheerful landlord and moderate social drinker, had a dangerous streak – and a peculiar interest in fire.

One customer remembered how he had been discussing with Arthur an atrocity that had featured in the newspapers and the landlord had explained that, if a body was properly burned by fire, no one could ever tell what had previously happened to it. It was, the publican remarked casually, a very easy thing to do.

As the day of their enforced departure from the pub drew nearer, life in the Bradbury household became more and more tense, although outwardly they did their best to keep up appearances. Maureen, four years older than her husband, a dainty, attractive blonde, was still her chirpy self behind the bar, Arthur dispensed his taproom philosophy unabated, and the two of them expressed confidence to anyone who would listen that they would get another pub.

But, inevitably, as each day went by and still they were not accepted anywhere else the pressure built. It was not just a matter of their livelihood but their home, their children's home. They were about to be cast out and, with each passing hour, the future looked more bleak.

On 16 June 1976, three days before they would have to leave, Arthur and Maureen had an interview for the position of steward and stewardess at the Enville Street Social Club in Ashton under Lyne. Neither was ever to discover that they had failed by just one vote to persuade the club committee that they were suitable. Indeed, when they returned to the pub that evening, they both appeared satisfied that the interview had gone supremely well and Arthur was certain that they had been successful. Maureen, typically, was rather more restrained.

Whatever their true feelings, within minutes of arriving back at Mother Mac's the couple began to row downstairs in front of the few customers still drinking. Although the landlord was aware that the Whitbread stocktaker was coming in the morning he had not banked the takings and Maureen let him know exactly what she thought of his lack of professionalism.

It may be that Arthur had already hatched his dark plot, in which case it was not surprising that when he finally closed the pub's doors the mood was less than pleasant.

At 7.30 the next morning, drayman John Gamett parked his wagon outside the pub, jumped down from the cab and pressed the doorbell. He always came early as Mother Mac's was in a narrow street in one of the busiest parts of the city and he liked to avoid the traffic.

Arthur Bradbury, who by this time had murdered his first four victims, opened the door almost immediately and treated his visitor to a deceptive smile.

The two men went to the cellar, where the publican pointed out which two tanks he had prepared to accept the delivery. The driver passed Arthur the valve, returned to his wagon, waited an appropriate few moments for the attachment to be secured and then turned on the pump, sending 180 gallons of beer rushing noisily down the tube.

The men chatted amicably over a freshly made pot of coffee while the beer tanks gurgled until they were full. Then, job done, the driver retracted his hoses and the delivery note was duly signed. If it had not been for the growing traffic the drayman might have thought about staying a little longer, carrying on the conversation, having another cup of coffee upstairs. Fortunately for him, he was diligent about his tasks of the morning, was happy to accept the gift of a packet of cigarettes proffered by the landlord and left. Alive.

A little earlier, as usual, Ann Hennegan, a family friend, had arrived to clean for the Bradburys. She wasn't paid but just did it to help out since she was so fond of Maureen.

Ann's husband was later to say how he thought Arthur was 'sly', how he didn't trust him and didn't like his boasting about being a former Commando schooled in unarmed combat. Mr Hennegan insisted he had been worried about Arthur for some time.

It is interesting to note how so many murderers, generally considered good company before they are exposed as killers, become, after the fact, suspicious-looking, shifty oddballs, obviously different. Weirdos.

Have you noticed how so many of history's famous killers have those distinctive staring eyes? Note the similarity between the Yorkshire Ripper, Peter Sutcliffe, and Charles Manson, the devil-worshipping monster who coordinated the Sharon Tate murders. Can you not actually see through those dark pupils into an evil, pitiless void where their souls should be? The answer is, actually, no, you can't.

I can't speak for Manson but Sutcliffe was by all accounts a most unremarkable man physically, a completely unprepossessing character who would never merit a second glance. At least, not until his bearded face was spread all over the front pages of the newspapers under headlines that suggested he was evil incarnate.

It is not difficult to stare at such a picture and become transfixed like a rabbit in a car's headlights. In these days of video and living colour the still photograph, especially in black and white, can be a thing of singular power. Often the picture the newspapers use is a mug shot taken at a police station after the individual concerned has spent hours or days being interrogated about their appalling crimes, not only getting very little sleep but also being forced to confront, often for the first time, the horror of their own actions, forced to see themselves as others do.

The visage that faces the lens is slack-lipped, deeply lined, hollow-eyed, with no trace of humour, cheerless in the extreme. A trick of the camera adds to the malevolent expression when a disembodied jailer's voice from behind the arc lights says flatly: 'Look straight ahead into the camera.' As the suspect obeys, too exhausted to care, raising their weary head, their eyelids lift but the eyes focus on nothing, the gaze going past the camera, searching for the photographer behind but not seeing anything. The shutter clicks, capturing the illuminated eyeball focused, not like in happy holiday snaps on the lens but much further back, appearing somehow to be staring insolently, dangerously out of the photograph.

The truth is that ninety-nine per cent of the time killers are just like the rest of us: thin, fat, tall, short, smart, scruffy, attractive or plain. It is not what they look like that sets them apart, it is what they do. Like us all, they have their ups and downs. The 'down' suffered by Arthur Bradbury, however, became a terminal free fall that needed a complex forensic examination to unravel.

As I was leaving the Manchester coroner's court an hour or so after Mrs Hennegan had been seen arriving at Mother Mac's, I was nearly run over by a fire engine speeding out of the firestation, which at that time was in the same building.

Two hours later, after attending another inquest in Oldham, I became reacquainted with the fire crew. They had been called to the pub after a typist in an overlooking office had noticed smoke coming out of the upper windows. One team of firemen, who were on the scene within four minutes of the 999 call, smashed through the locked front door while a second used a ladder to clamber through a second-floor window.

The building was full of dense smoke and the men all needed to wear breathing apparatus as they searched for the source of the fire and for any survivors who might be trapped in the various rooms. There were two main starting points of the fire, one in the cellar and another, much more intense, in a small storage room on the first floor. Both were quickly extinguished with powerful jets of water.

The crews searched the entire pub, finding a dead dog in one room and a dead cat in another, but no sign of people. Clothing was scattered around the smoke-filled main bedroom where the wardrobe and drawers had been left open.

When they reached the first floor, the storeroom blaze was immediately obvious to the firefighters, with flames visible at the top of the door, dancing brightly across the beam. The door opened outward and, as they pulled it, they were faced with what looked like a solid wall of furnace-like conflagration. Their water jet doused the flames, sending up clouds of steam, and remnants of black, burnt material floated in the hot air.

It was still difficult to see. The room housed the base of a dumb waiter that served the top two floors and had acted as a chimney for the fire, allowing the flames access to the upper rooms and feeding the fire with more oxygen. When the hoses had done their work, dealing with the main blaze, there were still two small, stuttering sources of flame in the room and a fireman went to deal with them. A blackened object, waist high, was blocking his way. It was a few moments before his trained, experienced eye realized the charred mass was a human body. At that point he backed out, touching nothing, knowing the rules.

He could not have been aware at that stage that the tiny cupboard-like room actually contained the remains of six people: Mr and Mrs Bradbury, their three children and Mrs Hennegan, the volunteer cleaner.

The dead were in a pile, one on top of the other, like soft logs, in what was effectively a family funeral pyre. All had been burned beyond the remotest possibility of recognition.

Uppermost was a male, lying on his back, facing up to the wrecked chute of the dumb waiter. There was something across the mouth that could have been a gag and the hands were tied behind his back with fabric, some of which had survived the heat.

Beneath him, only a leg showing until the removal of the first body, lay the second corpse, also gagged and bound, but this time with the hands held behind the back with wire. The body was bigger and it was female.

Below her was a second male. He was lying head down, close to the front of the dumb waiter, and there was no sign of any gag or binding.

The fourth body was a girl child, her left arm was bent behind her back as if it had been tied but there was no sign of what might have held it there. There was no obvious gag.

Next was an adult woman with wire around her right wrist and right ankle. She had been tied both hand and foot and also gagged with some sort of material.

Finally, at the bottom of the pile, lay another child, this time a boy, lying on his back, his hands tied behind his back with cloth.

Around and among them were items of clothing and a number of cushions and newspapers, all easily combustible material clearly placed there to assist the fire.

Examination of the floor of the room recovered from the ash a keyring with fourteen keys, two of Maureen Bradbury's rings, a cigarette lighter, a small padlock used to lock the storeroom and some coins in the remains of a cash drawer, similar to that in a shop's till.

I was also shown the bodies of an Alsatian dog in a bathroom on the second-floor landing and of a cat in a second-floor lounge. Autopsies on them showed they had died from the fumes created by the fire.

Once the positions of the human bodies had been carefully logged they were all taken in plastic bags to the Manchester mortuary less than a mile away.

I started with body number one.

It was that of a male child, about thirteen years old. There was a gag across the mouth and the internal organs showed signs associated with asphyxia. The most crucial factor here is the appearance of a number of small petechial haemorrhages on the surface of the heart. They are clear indications that the oxygen supply has been cut off, since that leads to the lining of blood vessels becoming damaged, rupturing and leaking blood. Normally, one would check for similar haemorrhages in the eyes but in this case they had been burned away. There was no evidence of carbon in the air passages or carbon monoxide in the blood, so this victim had stopped breathing before the fire had started and had been suffocated to death, probably with the gag that was found across his mouth.

Body number two was female and dissection revealed there had been a fusion of the right knee joint. Medical records revealed that Mrs Hennegan had had an accident as a child and undergone an operation for the removal of her patella, or kneecap. Fabric was around the mouth, and two rings, later identified as hers, were on her left hand. Again, the internal organs showed signs of asphyxia and there had been a fracture of the superior horn of the left thyroid cartilage in the larynx. The air passages, as before, were clear of carbon and the blood was free of carbon monoxide. She also had not died in the fire: she had been strangled, the larynx fracture typical of the use of powerful force on the throat.

The third body was different. This was an adult male who wore a ring on the third finger of his left hand. The air passages contained carbon particles and there was heat blistering of the epiglottis. The blood contained eighteen per cent carbon monoxide, which is an appreciable level, indicating that this body, which was neither tied nor gagged, had been alive at the beginning of the fire. He had no other obvious injuries.

Body number four had suffered similarly to the first two. A female child of approximately six years, she had an impression mark on her neck, typically the result of a ligature strangulation. Asphyxial signs were present but there was no carbon in the air passages or carbon monoxide in the blood. She too had been strangled.

The fifth body was that of a woman about five feet tall. She had a bracelet on her right wrist and two rings on the marriage finger. She had eaten a cheese-and-onion pie shortly before she died and was the only victim to show any evidence of having recently had a meal. Again, there were signs of asphyxia and she also had died before the fire began.

The sixth and final body corresponded to a boy child of about eleven. There was a ligature mark around the neck, a fracture of the thyroid bone and the tell-tale asphyxial signs. He too had died before the flames had got to him.

So, five of the bodies had been suffocated or strangled with ligatures before the fire. One, the third found, had been neither strangled nor tied up and had died instead from breathing in the fumes from the blaze.

The teeth from the first body were examined by forensic odontologist Dr J. Ken Holt, who compared dental records, matching them up with treatment received by Maureen's thirteen-year-old son Andrew.

The teeth in body number two had been neglected but corresponded to those of a woman of fifty. This, together with the jewellery and the deformity of the knee, identified Mrs Hennegan.

The Army dental history of Arthur Bradbury confirmed him as body number three.

Body number four was that of a little girl of approximately the age of Arthur's and Maureen's six-year-old daughter, Alison. There were no adequate dental records and nothing else identifiable on the body but, bearing in mind the whole scenario, we were prepared to accept the circumstantial evidence that this was Alison.

Body number five was that of a woman of between thirty-five and thirty-eight years of age with no significant dental abnormalities. But the jewellery and general development were sufficient to tell us this was Maureen.

The sixth and final body was confirmed by his school dental records as that of eleven-year-old James, Maureen's other son.

Detective Superintendent Jack Ridgway, head of

CID for the city centre, was now satisfied that he knew who was who in that home-made crematorium. But he still had to decide how they had got there.

My evidence showed that they had all died before they had been consumed by the fire, apart from Arthur Bradbury. So, with the pub doors locked from within and no sign of forced entry or exit, he had to be the chief suspect. But his body had itself been buried under two others. How could that have happened if he had killed them?

The blaze had raged with such intensity because of the chimney effect of the dumb waiter and the amount of material packed around the bodies, much of it obviously taken from the bedroom where the drawers and wardrobe had been left open. Someone had wanted that fire to be powerful.

Ridgway was soon made aware of the landlord's remarks about how burning a body can prevent anyone discovering what had happened to it and this increased the detective's suspicions about Arthur. The publican appeared to have been suggesting that, if a fire was sufficiently intense, absolutely everything could be destroyed to the extent that forensic examination of the scene would be worthless, all the clues gone.

If so, he was wrong. This fire was certainly very severe and had probably been burning for several minutes even before the smoke was noticed outside, and the bodies were undeniably badly damaged. But still there was plenty for us to go at.

The evidence piled up against Bradbury; he was known to have been violent towards his wife, he had been under pressure because of being forced to leave the pub, he had previously made an attempt at arson, and he had been the last to die, the only one killed by the fire. But how did bodies, already dead, come to bury him?

The answer was in the dumb waiter.

My tests suggested that Maureen, probably the first to die, had been killed soon after eating her pie, possibly as early as 1.00 a.m., six hours or more before the drayman was greeted so warmly.

Mrs Hennegan, the last to be murdered, was seen alive at 9.05 a.m. sweeping the footpath outside Mother Mac's. Just five minutes later a stocktaker from the Whitbread Brewery had arrived to check on the untrustworthy publican but had got no response. The cleaner was in the habit of taking tea and toast with Mrs Bradbury in the upstairs living quarters after she had completed her tasks. Clearly, she would not have found her friend in her usual place and there could be little doubt that when the stocktaker called she was either dead or dying.

Interestingly, Arthur, a cold killing machine by this stage, had chosen to let the drayman go and he may have attempted to persuade Mrs Hennegan to leave unmolested before she saw something she shouldn't. He might have told her his wife was out or ill or busy. He might have wanted to spare this kindly lady. Or he might have killed her without compunction, without worry or concern, already too steeped in blood to be bothered about taking yet another innocent life.

In the event Mrs Hennegan was probably caught from behind with the ligature, which was pulled tight and held until she died, the fabric placed in her mouth after her breathing stopped.

The night before the carnage Arthur and Maureen had been arguing in front of customers and it is entirely possible that their row continued and became worse. The children would have been in bed by that time, either asleep or listening to the adults shouting at each other.

Ridgway concluded that Maureen had been the first victim, strangled in a rage. But instead of that horror sating Bradbury's lust for violence, the dreadful event merely supplied the momentum for the systematic murder of his entire family.

Killing one's wife in blind anger is one thing, going from room to room intent on killing children is entirely another. Bradbury's behaviour was almost unbelievably savage.

Establishing precise timings was not possible so it is unclear whether Bradbury left Maureen immediately to continue the slaughter or first carried her down the stairs to the storeroom before visiting the children. We cannot tell whether he agonized over what to do next or proceeded without pause, without mercy. It is not impossible that one of the youngsters came in, saw what had happened and started screaming. A simple choke hold around the neck may have seemed the best way for a man fresh from killing to stifle quickly the intruding, infuriating sound.

There were no signs of a struggle in any of the bedrooms so it would appear that whatever Bradbury did he did efficiently. Of course, if he had come into their rooms there would have been no need for any of them to be worried, no need to be concerned if Daddy touched them, not even if he held their throats.

A man of reasonable fitness and average strength would be able to dispatch children of that age and build very quickly. Bradbury had told friends he was trained in unarmed combat. It had been his proud boast.

The leap from loving father to killer of children is one that can surely only be made when all normal reactions, feelings, emotions and sensibilities have been placed in suspension. We must also consider the matter of the bonds used to tie the victims' arms and legs. Normally one would not tie up the dead, there would be little point. So, assuming that they were alive while trussed up, what kind of terror was visited upon them as they were dispatched one by one? The mother, then the children, either too scared or too trusting to scream. How long did this last? How long did they live, knowing that they were about to die? Can children ever, whatever the extreme circumstances, comprehend that they are about to have their lives extinguished by the man they call 'father'? And if they can is that not the most appalling outrage of all?

This is a far stride from rational behaviour. If Bradbury had survived, I suspect a plea of insanity would not have been contested too strongly by the prosecution.

It took time, certainly, for Bradbury to build his human bonfire. His first task had been to carry a mattress from one of the bedrooms and place it on the floor of the storeroom. On that, face up, he placed the body of James, the younger of Maureen's two sons by her previous marriage.

What would Bradbury have seen when he studied

the child's still face? Would he even have recognized the boy? Upon him he placed the youngster's mother, his own wife. Their heads were close together. Around them both he packed tightly pieces of clothing and papers, shoving incendiary material between the bodies like sandwich fillings.

On top of them Bradbury placed Alison, the daughter he and Maureen had created together. Slightly built even for a six-year-old, she was on her back, her left arm pulled unnaturally behind her by her bonds, her fair hair, soon to be burned away, falling to one side, away from her pale face.

That mound of bodies would have reached a level roughly in line with the entrance gate of the dumb waiter. Andrew, the older of the two boys, was bent at his hip and curled up into the left-hand carriage of the wooden hoist that had for years served the building, running between floors on a sturdy rope. It was only twenty-one inches square at the base and three feet high but it had been large enough to take him.

It is thought this whole macabre task of carrying and stacking bodies would have taken at least an hour and would have been very hard work. What time he began is a matter of conjecture. But it seems he had finished and had made a fresh pot of coffee by the time the drayman, Mr Gamett, arrived in the morning with his delivery. Arthur, people remembered, looked composed but tired and his hair had not been combed.

Once the dray had left and while Mrs Hennegan was still busy with her cleaning, the landlord went down into the cellar and carried out a last, petty act of vengeance against the brewery, opening valves on the beer tanks and pouring 480 gallons of ale worth nearly £1,000 down the drain.

That process would have taken nearly an hour and that Bradbury should have left his wife's friend upstairs while he was doing it suggests that either he had a lot of nerve or he was past caring. Whatever was his initial plan, by 9.10 a.m., Mrs Hennegen was dead by his hand.

Bradbury carried her body into the storeroom, used the pulley to raise the cage that held Andrew's bent form and placed her underneath it, head first, in the space it left at the bottom of the dumb waiter.

Later police found a large suitcase in the cellar. It was packed with Embassy and Benson and Hedges cigarettes, six bottles of Scotch and two of Southern Comfort. In the bedroom was a plastic salt box containing £279. It is possible Arthur was planning to take these items with him but nowhere did investigators find a case of clothing. If the man was intending to start a fire and disappear, hoping that the bodies would disintegrate completely and the police suspect he was among the dead, one would have expected him to take clothes.

It is impossible to know which of the two fires, upstairs and down, was started first. But both were burning when Arthur Bradbury found himself in the storeroom, looking at his obscene handiwork: his wife, his two stepsons, his own tiny daughter and a woman he called a friend, all dead because of his own inadequacies, their faces twisted by the strangulation, their protruding tongues pushing with a repulsive leer at the thin fabric of the gags.

Perhaps he had a glimpse of sanity, was confronted

by the evil he had done and saw only one way out. Who knows?

The detective was, nevertheless, certain of one thing. As the flames licked around his family, as the pungent smell of burning flesh reached his nostrils, Arthur Bradbury, quietly spoken, easygoing, one of the lads, pulled the door of the tiny room closed behind him and threw himself, alive, on to the blistering remains of those he had once loved.

The fire grew quickly, feeding on the body fat now leaking from the corpses and the fresh air from the dumb-waiter shaft. Soon the rope holding Andrew's cage was burning and splitting until it separated, dropping the wooden box on to Mrs Hennegan's body.

A short time later the wooden base of the hoist was itself reduced to ashes and the bodies of the boy and the woman tumbled out on top of the man who was now damned by his own hellfire.

Three weeks before Christmas in 1974, an eighteen-year-old machine operator called Alec Beech clambered up a drainpipe outside a well-kept council house on a pleasant estate and shimmied through a small window that had been left open.

It was his older brother Roy's house and no one had seen the twenty-four-year-old painter and decorator, his wife or their three children for more than a month.

When the teenager got inside, it quickly became clear that the placid exterior of the unobtrusive little home hid a scene of appalling devastation. In room after room, nearly everything that could be broken had been smashed into pieces in what was obviously some kind of vented fury or terrible frustration. Nearly all the family's possessions had been systematically destroyed in a sustained act of wilful vandalism.

Curiously, among the wreckage of broken crockery, glass, furniture and ripped carpet, a few items, mostly fairly new, remained unscathed, still neatly tidied away. We were later to discover that Roy Beech was nothing if not neat.

He was in bed, his left arm draped around his wife, his left hand with a wedding band on the appropriate finger resting on her chest and his face nuzzling against her cheek. In the same double divan, tucked, like their parents, under a purple quilt and a cream eiderdown and wearing their nightclothes, were the couple's son and two daughters.

The elder girl, Samantha Jane, aged five, lay closest to her father, facing his back. Next to her was three-year-old Kelly, and the only boy, John, aged seven, was on the outside, the far right looking from the foot of the bed.

Like their sister, both John and Kelly lay on their right sides, facing their dad.

Among this group of five recumbent figures in a perfectly ordinary suburban bedroom, with orange flowers on the wallpaper and a clock by the bed, only the mother, Demrhys, twenty-seven, whom all her friends and neighbours called Debbie, lay on her left.

Their eyes were all clogged with brown fungal growths, a typical sign that suggested to me on first viewing that they had been dead for several weeks. Given enough time, settling spores will develop abundantly if they are left undisturbed in relatively warm temperatures on an appropriate growth medium.

On closer inspection I saw that the lumpy collections of live matter beginning to extend down Roy's face were much more pronounced than on the others. It occurred to me that this greater proliferation might have been because he had been crying before he slipped into his fatal sleep. Fungi like the damp.

Roy had died from barbiturate poisoning after taking a large amount of a fast-acting sleeping tablet called Tuinol – which is now no longer prescribed, not least because of its potentially dangerous strength.

Toxicology tests on blood and urine samples showed quantities of the drug well beyond overdose levels and residue of the tablets Roy had taken was recovered from the stomach. There were no marks of violence on the body nor signs of internal injuries that could have contributed to his death. He had been a healthy young man.

A similar fate had befallen his two daughters. Both Samantha Jane and Kelly had died after taking pills that, to them, would have looked like sweets and were sugar-coated. As the formula was sufficiently powerful to knock out most adults within minutes, the effect upon small children would have been extremely swift. These little girls would have been unconscious within ten minutes at most and dead within the hour. It would not have been necessary for them to swallow more than half a dozen tablets each.

Things were different with the son, John. There was obvious bruising on the right side of his neck, both inside and out, and haemorrhages in his eyes and on the surface of his heart. These are classic signs of stran-gulation. He had not taken any significant amount of barbiturate and I concluded that he had died at the hands of another, literally.

Mrs Beech, too, had been killed by means other than poison. Demrhys had some old bruises and a tattoo on her left forearm but nothing significant became apparent until I began an examination of her back. There was a small incised wound, four-fifths of an inch across, between the seventh and eighth ribs. An instrument had entered here and been pushed into the thoracic cavity. This would not have taken a great deal of force as it only had to pass through the soft cartilage between the ribs rather than break through any hard bone. The cartilage is the substance that allows the ribcage to expand and contract as we breathe and is, of necessity, relatively non-resistant. A sharp knife can pass through it easily.

A feature of knife attacks is that, purely by luck, a savage assault can result in relatively minor damage if the assailant's blade is deflected by a hard rib and prevented from entering the danger area. But a soft, even half-hearted lunge can result in a murder charge if the instrument finds a place where only cartilage is protecting the heart, lungs and major vessels.

In this case Mrs Beech had been extremely unfortunate in that the weapon used had slipped easily into her chest but had avoided all the danger areas – except one. It had just nicked the main descending aorta, causing a tiny cut but a lethal one. If the blade had been half a millimetre to one side or had travelled half a millimetre less deeply into her chest she would have lived. As it was, blood began to drip through the tissue of the aorta, at first only in minuscule amounts. But as the pressure from the beating heart continued remorse-lessly, pumping seventy or so times a minute, the tiny hole became bigger and the outcome inevitable.

Demrhys would not have known she was dying and would have been unlikely to have been in much pain, the only such feeling coming from the skin damage caused by the small incision made by the blade. Tiredness is the most she would probably have felt. But eventually, suddenly, the wall of the aorta would have burst and death would have followed in moments.

If she had been conscious when it happened it would have come as a complete surprise.

The Beech family had lived for several years in the house in Micklehurst Green, Offerton, Stockport, and were well liked by the locals who told how Roy and his wife were clearly devoted to each other. However it seems that both of them were significantly flawed psychologically.

Debbie was adopted, spoiled by her adoptive parents and started to steal as a child. She was arrested for theft the night she married Roy, but the magistrate took pity on her because it was Christmas and let her out.

Her husband was born with two teeth, which was said to be a lucky sign, but they were taken out in case he swallowed them. At the age of eleven his father got him drunk as a joke. His mother didn't see the funny side and strapped him into a pram until he sobered up.

Soon he was playing truant with his father's approval. They were close, spending a lot of time together, and Roy, a big lad who looked older than his years, developed a taste for beer at an early age.

Debbie, three years older, set her sights on the tough young man. They married when he was just sixteen, conniving to get parental approval by claiming falsely that she was pregnant and they had no choice. But in any case Roy was a father by seventeen with the arrival of John.

Before Samantha Jane was born, Debbie had a miscarriage and started taking tablets for depression. She was to continue taking them in varying strengths and combinations for the next six years, until she died.

Roy hated Debbie's growing dependence on the drugs that, it was said, sometimes plunged her into a zombie-like state, and violent arguments would take place. But his wife's family have always argued that he had a naturally vicious streak and used her addiction merely as the excuse he needed to hit her. Their relationship was undoubtedly stormy, but they always made up after their rows.

The couple spent money well beyond their means and became heavily in debt, with Roy eventually being declared bankrupt. Illogically, the spending went on, based on the theory that so far only one of them was bankrupt and they could carry on until it happened to the other. Pressure squeezed hard on all sides.

When Roy's teenage brother climbed through the window of their house he found one apologetic suicide note addressed to Debbie's adoptive father and another, with more specific details about what had happened, addressed to the police. There was also a wallet containing £54 neatly set aside to cover funeral expenses.

The letters explained that, during a row over

Debbie's drug taking, Roy had demanded to know where she had hidden her tablets but she had refused to tell him. He had threatened her with a sheath knife but still she would not tell.

Samantha, the note read, had declared that she knew the pills' whereabouts. She had offered to tell her father, at which point her mother had hit the youngster five times on the head with a bottle. It was at that moment, Roy Beech claimed, that he had lunged forward with the knife.

It was not much of a wound, he thought, and Debbie went to bed alone. About four hours later he went up and discovered she was 'unwell'.

The letter went on: 'I can't live without Demrhys. I don't want the children in a home or someone else bringing them up. I hope God will forgive me for what I have done. I love them all. Please try to keep us together.'

Whether Roy was telling the whole truth or not I cannot know, although I did not find any significant wound on Samantha's head. But it would seem likely that most of his account was accurate. The lunge with the knife would have ended any discussion, each party for their own reasons wanting an end to the arguing at that point.

Roy Beech, angry and perhaps dismayed at his own action, would have quietened down after the sudden surge of adrenalin accompanying the attack. Although Debbie would have been shocked at the realization she had been stabbed, she would almost certainly have had the strength to walk upstairs unaided and get into bed.

Roy's discovery of her, probably already dead, some

hours later, precipitated an action that many, including myself, find it difficult to understand or forgive.

It seems that the two girls were persuaded easily enough to take the pills. They would have trusted their father. But the boy, at seven years of age the oldest child, was strangled. This suggests that the youngster was reluctant to follow the same path as his sisters and Roy took it on himself to throttle his own son with his own hands. In his letter he said he would kill them all with tablets so they would die peacefully. Often, it appears, when a person takes a violent road, the path can dip with alarming speed, tumbling the individual into unfathomable depths.

Once his family was dead, Roy Beech went around the house with some kind of blunt instrument, furiously and yet methodically trashing his life, his history, everything he had become, to smithereens. But he went about it in an obsessively neat fashion. He smashed everything that was paid for but left untouched any item on which he still owed money. Nothing on HP was even marked. That terrible day he destroyed only that which he considered his own, bought and paid for.

At the last, his destructive energy spent, Roy laid the three feather-light, lifeless bodies in the bed alongside their mother's now-cold corpse. He took time to arrange the boy and two girls in a neat line, all facing the same way, on their sides as if asleep. Then, having already swallowed the lethal sleeping draught, he climbed between his children and wife to join them in death.

Closing his eyes against the abject sorrow that was welling up uncontrollably, Roy held the woman he loved in a final embrace. His regretful, bitter tears spilled wet on his cheeks, which were soon to host another, lower form of life.

4

Mr Asia

You don't really get a lot of laughs in my job, but I had to smile at the handless corpse.

This poor fellow had been through a lot. He had been shot twice in the head, both his hands had been chopped off and were missing, his face had been bludgeoned, smashing several teeth and fracturing his nose and jaw, and he had been stabbed in the abdomen before being thrown naked into a flooded quarry with weights tied to his body.

The only clue to his identity was a Chinese medallion around his neck. The police took it to a local Chinese chip shop, hoping someone might be able to decipher the mysterious symbol.

An old man at the shop recognized the ancient sign at once. It meant: Good Luck and Long Life!

On the day, I have to admit, I thought this was hilarious. I had never seen a man more dead and the only clue the police had to go on wished him well. However, as time has passed and certain events have occurred involving the people who were responsible for this, I have wondered about the mystical powers of that gold pendant and why these thorough and professional killers failed to remove it from their victim's body.

Initially, it seemed they had done their job very well. I had the feeling they had done this kind of thing before. The actual killing had been carried out with two bullets in the brain at contact range. They had tied his legs together with blue nylon cord, which was in turn attached to four weights, two of 14 1bs and two of 56 1bs. Another cord had been wrapped around his neck and both arms and tied to a green motor jack.

His abdomen had been slashed open, not for any gratuitous reason but to allow the gases that would be formed during the putrefaction of the body to escape, thus preventing him from blowing up like a balloon and rising to the surface of the flooded quarry.

The hands had been removed because he had a criminal record and could have been traced by his fingerprints. His face had been smashed in to hamper any dental or photographic identification in the unlikely event of him ever being found.

The chances were that he would have remained at the bottom of that deep, dark pool until the water and the living things in it had completed the natural decaying process: the tissues reducing and joining the silt, the bones becoming covered in tangled, camouflaging weed, the metal weights sinking into the soft mud.

The killers' added advantage was that their victim had been the sort of man whose lifestyle meant he could vanish without warning at practically any time. There would have been no missing person's report, so no investigation and consequently no risk of capture.

It could have been the perfect crime. But luck deserted them.

Their first bit of bad fortune was that, as the body sank, one of the nylon lines snagged on some submerged growth and the corpse stayed much closer to the surface than they'd intended. Secondly, they couldn't have known that the Lancashire Police Underwater Search Unit used that very spot for training.

Five days after the killing, divers practising their techniques in the murky water spotted a pale figure that they thought at first was a tailor's dummy. But when one of the scuba team got close enough to touch it he suddenly found himself needing fresh air fast.

Instead of disappearing without trace, the handless corpse was headline news within days. Its discovery triggered one of the biggest manhunts this country has seen, stretching into Asia and Australia as detectives got on the trail of a villainous and hugely wealthy drugs syndicate.

Eventually, the principals in this horrific murder were caught, tried and jailed. The main culprit later paid the ultimate price when he collapsed and died in mysterious circumstances in prison.

He had defied the odds for years and had made a fortune out of his ruthless criminal activities. But the day he ordered the murder of a man who wore an Oriental good-luck symbol, his own luck ran out.

I would not have become involved at all except that, on the day the body was found at a place called Heskin Delph, near Chorley, on a Sunday morning in October 1979, my colleague, Dr Brian Beeson, who would normally have covered that patch, was attending another case in Carlisle.

When I arrived in the late afternoon, the police frogmen were still having difficulty getting the body out of the water. But within an hour they had managed to move it and the weights onto a small sandy area. It was steep and difficult to get down so it was decided to move the dead man to the mortuary at Preston Royal Infirmary. At 7.30 p.m. the examination began.

Both hands had been amputated at the wrist. The edges of the cuts were rough and showed no evidence of vital reaction, suggesting the hands had been removed, probably with a small axe, after death had occurred. The right wrist had three adjacent superficial cuts and had been severed through the lower end of the radius and ulna. The left had been cut across the lower end of the ulna and through the proximal carpal joint.

There were seven ragged wounds running vertically on the abdomen through which loops of small intestine were protruding. One of the powerful upward sweeps with the sharp instrument used had risen sufficiently high to cause bruising on the lower ribs.

There was a puncture mark, which was blackened around the edges, about half an inch in diameter and two inches in front of the right ear. This was a bullet-entry wound. A small exit wound was found at the same spot on the other side of his head. Someone had held a gun close against the victim's temple on the right side and had shot straight through his brain.

A second entry wound was found at the back of the head but the bullet had not exited. A track showed it to be still inside his skull, having come to rest on the right wing of the sphenoid bone. One bullet had killed him, the second had made absolutely certain. It was cold-blooded in the extreme.

As with the wrists, the injuries to the front of the head and face showed little evidence of reaction. I concluded that they, together with the abdominal wounds, had been caused after death.

Two weeks later a beautiful young woman walked into

the police station at Chorley where the investigation was in full cry but getting nowhere and told detectives that she had been away in Spain but had read about the murder on her return. She identified the body as that of her boyfriend, New Zealander Marty Johnstone, who had been a very handsome, very successful and extremely rich international drug smuggler.

From that moment the inquiry took on an unprecedented scope, with British officers travelling to Singapore, New Zealand, Australia and the United States. Information, backed up by statements from witnesses, many of whom were given remarkable levels of round-the-clock personal protection, was gathered from all four corners of the earth and filtered back to the somewhat unlikely nerve centre in rainswept Lancashire.

Once it began to come in, the stream of facts and figures turned into a torrent. Johnstone, it became clear, was at least the twelfth person to have been murdered in a short space of time by the ruthless drugs gang in which he was himself a major figure. People who had information on the smugglers and their operations were suddenly terrified that they would be next to be murdered and fell over each other to try to help the police lock up the killer.

Johnstone had been considered one of the elite untouchables. If he could be killed then, clearly, no one was safe.

The twenty-nine-year-old playboy had started out as a second-rate crook in his home country where, while in jail, he had met another small-time hood called Alexander Sinclair who had dabbled in narcotics. They became partners in petty crime but soon realized their endeavours would never satisfy the gnawing ambition both had for the high life.

They moved into drugs in a relatively minor fashion, buying cannabis from Thai sailors who hid small amounts on board fishing vessels and container ships. But in 1975 the pair decided to go for broke and ploughed their so-far-meagre profits into personally running a series of cannabis-smuggling trips between Thailand and Auckland in a small, rickety speedboat. They risked everything in treacherous waters patrolled both by lawmen and vicious pirates, but they made it.

Their success produced sufficient funds for Johnstone to buy a larger vessel, a twenty-metre yawl called the *Brigadoon*. Late in their inaugural year they avoided a Customs trap and landed 400,000 cannabis sticks worth £2 million.

Suddenly they were rich. They had enough money to retire into a life of luxury. But they showed a trait common to most crooks: they got greedy. Like the gambler who wins first time, they couldn't believe how easy it was and they saw no reason to slow down.

Sinclair set up business fronts in Australia and New Zealand while Johnstone launched a company in Singapore breeding tropical fish for export. They soon had businesses dealing in anything from live alligators to cane furniture and billiard tables, all providing the necessary legitimate cover for Johnstone to arrange and supervise the purchase of heroin and cocaine, drugs that have much higher profit margins than cannabis.

He travelled extensively, slipping easily into the life to which he had always aspired, and set up an extravagant home and luxury offices in Singapore. Soon he was known by underworld contacts as 'Mr Asia'. He relished the name.

Always wearing a silk shirt and bedecked in heavy

jewellery, Johnstone insisted his favourite drink was Dom Perignon champagne. He flew on the inaugural Concorde flight from Singapore to London where his land transport was a chauffeur-driven Jaguar.

Women found him and his money irresistible and he had no trouble finding willing volunteers among his glamorous conquests to act as couriers, taking extraordinary risks to carry drugs through Customs. In the Far East, the law often implemented a mandatory death sentence for those caught.

It is difficult to work out how Johnstone could develop such a hold on the women that they would put their lives on the line for him. Although they received lavish gifts and his occasional attentions, they were paid comparatively tiny amounts of cash for taking staggering risks. I can only imagine that they were 'risk groupies', high on the excitement that the man, his cash, his style and his danger provided. That they trusted his judgement so totally is a testimony to his powers of persuasion.

A single trip could bring in heroin or 'coke' worth £1.5 million on the streets of Melbourne, most of which was clear profit for the now well-established duo. Much of this was reinvested back into the business, doubling, trebling and quadrupling profits with each fresh trip.

Sinclair, five years older than his friend, used his new-found liquidity to develop the organization and establish new branches in Fiji, the US and Britain, and to bribe police, Customs officers and lawyers to ensure he stayed one step ahead of the authorities.

It cost him around £10,000 a year to acquire a good insider. He tapped phones and used vast sums of money to employ new-technology communication systems to keep his own operation tight as a drum.

Sinclair recognized that it was smart, as in any business, not to waste profits but to use them to improve the operation for the future. He was brighter than Marty and, it transpired, a lot nastier, too.

The organization became increasingly sophisticated and daring, developing a method of encasing drugs in 'dog-proof' glass-fibre blocks so they could not be sniffed out. In just nine months 48 kilos of heroin worth just under £50 million was imported into Australia, mostly from Thailand and the Philippines.

Just two years out of petty theft and thuggery, Sinclair boasted proudly that he could never spend the interest on his newly amassed fortune, let alone the capital.

Like Johnstone, he gained a taste for fast cars and women. But he also developed a reputation as a hard man. Some knew him as 'The Ace', others as 'The Australian Jackal'. As his power grew and he established control of the drugs market in that part of the world, the narcotics and homicide squads in Australia found their overtime bills going up.

The skeleton of 'Pommy' Harry Lewis, a small-time dealer, was found in a shallow grave in New South Wales. Someone had cut off his hands at the wrists. A courier, Maria Hisshion, was found floating in Sydney Harbour, shot dead.

Police have information that the corpses of two more, Greg Ollard and Julie Theilman, are under a section of the concrete that makes up one of the runways at Sydney Airport. Sinclair was getting kill crazy. Anyone who crossed him – or even anyone he *thought* had crossed him – was in serious trouble.

One of his paid contacts in the Australian police tipped

him off that two couriers, a married couple called Douglas and Isobel Wilson, were secretly spilling their story to the drugs squad. The pair had been taken on by Sinclair to replace the people he'd had buried at the airport but, unfortunately, they had become aware of their predecessors' unpleasant fate, lost their nerve completely and run to the authorities.

They told of massive drug deals, clandestine meetings, secret drops, threats and beatings. They named leading members of a criminal outfit known simply as The Organization. And they spoke of murder. Sections of their taped police interviews were copied by bent cops in Sinclair's employ and delivered to him, and from that moment the Wilsons were doomed.

Five months before the handless corpse in the Chorley quarry on the other side of the world was discovered, an inquisitive Antipodean dog called Mitzi scratched at a patch of soil in Rye, Sydney, and uncovered what was left of Douglas and Isobel, badly decomposed, lying on top of each other and covered with less than three feet of damp sand. Both had been shot in the head and had been dead for about a month.

The police investigators found a woman witness who started to tell all about a man she knew as Terence Clarke who, she claimed, was the all-powerful head of a major drugs syndicate. She had fallen in love with him but now, faced with his maniacal thirst for blood, she had become afraid and was prepared to spill everything.

It transpired that Clarke and Sinclair were one and the same man. 'Miss X' later became a key witness in the trial at Lancaster Crown Court when he was accused of the murder of his friend and partner in crime, Marty Johnstone.

The discovery of the bodies meant that Australia was suddenly a very hot place for The Organization and alternative accommodation was sought. Months earlier, Johnstone had travelled to the UK to look at prospects there. He had flown over with his 'first lieutenant', Andrew Maher, who, before emigrating to New Zealand, had been brought up in Lancashire.

Back at his roots, Maher worked as the English representative for Johnstone's companies, successfully fronting the outwardly legitimate offices that were the front for more smuggling. The set-up was secure, solid and prosperous, so when the time for a move suddenly arrived it seemed sensible that the centre of operations should be transferred to the UK and divided between Lancashire and London.

The two men had put together an impressive operation, recruiting a 'banker' to handle and launder cash, drivers, couriers and minders who knew how to use firearms. But while the rest of the gang had been busy dodging the police in Australia, Johnstone had been taking advantage somewhat.

Perhaps partly because he had taken to ingesting quite a lot of the expensive substances he was importing, his judgement was occasionally clouded. He started making mistakes, both in his smuggling activities and in his perception of his position within this volatile group. Lulled into buying a shipment of sugar when he expected cocaine, he cost the gang £750,000 and when one of his deals with suppliers in Thailand went wrong The Organization lost £500,000.

The profits were so huge that even these losses could have been written off. But Marty had been salting away a heavy percentage of the UK operation's cash into his personal accounts, and Sinclair believed that at least some of these apparent errors were not mistakes at all, but Johnstone skimming off the top.

Marty had also told his partner on several occasions that he disapproved of his tactics of extreme violence because such behaviour was likely to attract unwarranted police attention. This too angered Sinclair, who didn't take kindly to criticism. When he flew into Britain, using one of his many aliases, and based himself in a smart flat in Kensington, he already had a plan in mind.

Sinclair chose Marty's closest ally, the person he most trusted, his old friend Andrew Maher, to carry out the hit. Maher was informed that once Johnstone was dead he, Maher, would replace him as number two in The Organization. It was, as they say in these circles, an offer he couldn't refuse. Johnstone was told he was needed to set up a deal in Scotland and was picked up in London by Maher and two henchmen.

Their luxury Jaguar came to a halt at a lay-by on the A6 motorway near Lancaster, an area Maher knew well. He pulled a gun from his pocket, ordered Marty out of the car and shot him. The killers bundled the body into the boot, drove thirty miles to Maher's home in Leyland and parked up in the garage where Maher changed into a pair of overalls and took an axe and a hammer to his former friend's remains. After the body was dumped the hands were taken north and thrown into the River Almond in Scotland.

When Lancashire Police acted on the information supplied by Johnstone's girlfriend they soon had the men responsible for carrying out the murder and one explained what had happened to the hands. Police divers were sent to the river and discovered the dismembered right hand. The other, either washed away or picked up by some animal, was never recovered. But it didn't matter.

Twenty-five days after I carried out the post-mortem on the body in the quarry I was shown the hand at the North-Western Forensic Science Laboratory at Chorley.

The lower process of the ulna bone had been broken away from the stump of the right arm that I had viewed previously and was found in the recovered hand. X-ray pictures also perfectly matched the bones, like pieces from a jigsaw. The hand belonged to the dead man. Fingerprints later confirmed what police had been told by the witness: the handless corpse was drug runner Marty Johnstone.

The hand remained at the lab for several years, preserved in a jar, to be brought out for lectures and suchlike. The cold water in the river had kept it in reasonable condition before it was found and brought to Chorley. Unfortunately, air did get to it eventually. It became rather unpleasant and had to be disposed of.

Sinclair made it clear from the moment he was arrested that he had resources he intended to use to get him sprung from jail. He let it be known that his freedom was worth £1 million in cash money. Before his trial a rumour circulated that there was to be an attempt to break him out of Strangeways Jail in Manchester where he was being held on remand. Troops were secretly brought in but nothing happened.

Two years after his conviction, Sinclair claimed he was prepared to tell the authorities how laundered drug money had been used to buy weapons for the IRA. By a remarkable coincidence, a fortnight later he collapsed and died on his way to lunch at Parkhurst Jail on the Isle of Wight, apparently from a heart attack.

The authorities never did manage to trace The Organization's assets, stashed in various banks across the world. In December 1984, sixteen months after Sinclair's death, a New Zealand judge ruled the killer's last will and testament to be valid. It bequeathed his £30 million fortune to his son, Jarrod, then aged six, and stipulated that he should receive it when he reached the age of twenty-five. As the cash is outside Australian, New Zealand or UK jurisdiction, no one can stop him receiving it.

Now there's a piece of luck, as they say in the Orient.

5

Death as a Way of Life

Forty years ago a driver was very seriously injured in a crash at an accident black spot near the smart Mere Golf and Country Club, just outside Knutsford in Cheshire. Once the firemen had dug him out of what was left of his car, he was taken by ambulance to the nearest suitably equipped hospital, a small unit in Altrincham about five miles away where I was working in Casualty.

I had recently completed my year as a houseman and was at that early stage in my career where I was trying to decide which medical direction I wanted to take. I had already considered working in a laboratory to gain some general insight into medicine and on this occasion, as there was no on-call pathologist, I found myself having to group and cross-match the blood for the injured man who was about to have emergency surgery.

While I was giving him preliminary treatment I became aware of an odd, waxy smell. It was neither pleasant nor unpleasant, somewhere between furniture polish and old grease. The odour was not at first very pronounced but was growing stronger, lingering around the trolley on which the patient was laid. It almost had texture and possessed a strange kind of warmth that passed on heat but seemed somehow to bring about a change in temperature. It was, I knew instantly, the smell of death.

It became a familiar scent over the years. It was almost comforting in that, whenever it was around, even before I had seen the body in question or been supplied with details of the death, it confirmed the fact that I was on my 'territory'. That gave me a greater feeling of security.

Unfortunately, it was often accompanied by a second smell, that of decomposition. This has no such comforting feature, quite the reverse. It is possibly the most disgusting smell on earth. Depending on how much the bacteria affect the tissues concerned, it can be like a smack in the nose: you recoil as if someone has hit you with a cricket bat. It is as pungent as ammonia but then it sticks to the back of your throat and even seems to get into your ears.

When decomposition begins, the tissues very quickly start to go green. If you have a trained eye and don't absolutely have to hang around, one sight of the tell-tale colour is enough to send most experienced people scattering for air.

Until relatively modern times, we pathologists weren't helped much by the fact that the local authorities, whose responsibility it was to provide mortuaries, didn't rate this duty as a priority. Consequently, we regularly found ourselves working in little huts with no ventilation and no sluicing.

Some were thoughtfully situated near rivers, streams or canals so we at least had water with which to wash the place down afterwards. But, particularly in summer, the work could be hell. There were no fridges so we had to work fast.

I recall one coroner, Geoffrey Rothwell, walking into a small mortuary that rarely had more than one body in it, but on this day had two rather smelly cases. He went grey, took two steps back and declared with all the authority he could muster: 'This mortuary is condemned.'

On another occasion, at Middleton mortuary, I was dealing with a chap who was extremely bloated because of the gases being produced by the feeding bacteria in his gut. The people who had no choice but to be witnesses to the post-mortem would dash outside, breathe in large lungfuls of air and hold it for as long as possible before repeating the action. They were green, too.

Another rather unpleasant case was that of a man discovered in a field near Clatterbridge Hospital on the Wirral. He was easy to find because a line of creepy-crawlies was walking across the road back to where they had come from, after visiting his corpse. When we opened him up we found that most of his insides were gone, eaten by the maggots, but in the two inches of stomach that was left intact there was a quantity of barbiturates stuck to the wall. He had died from an overdose.

All this may lead you to feel that I made the wrong choice of profession, but not so. The man from the road accident was indeed close to death: he could not have been closer with the injuries he had sustained. The smell of death was upon him and I was convinced that he would not last the duration of the operation. But he did, and survived to leave the hospital and return to his family.

Death had been there in the room but had been forced away at the last possible moment, the patient dragged back from the edge. It had quite a profound effect on me.

Coincidentally, a pathologist who noticed my interest in the pathology side of the case informed me there was a vacancy for a resident pathologist at a hospital in Bolton, Lancashire. I felt that this was a rapidly expanding field of medicine that was going to increase in scope and importance and was bound to be fascinating. Its role in diagnosis and the monitoring of treatments was playing a more and more vital role, growing in usefulness with each improvement in medical technique and scientific knowledge. It seemed to me that this was where the action was. I applied and got the job.

Two years in Bolton were followed by National Service. I served as a pathologist in Northern Nigeria where tropical diseases kept me busy.

Further training in Lancaster and Manchester led to a consultancy at the Oldham group of hospitals where I remained until my retirement.

Throughout those years, I have constantly studied the cause of death. It has been my professional life and it is rare that I am unable to offer at least an informed opinion on what caused someone's demise.

That is, I can usually resolve the question 'How?' However, the answer to the question 'Why?' is more elusive.

We die, of course, when our bodies can no longer function, when certain vital components that make up the human form cease to operate correctly and their contribution to the working of the whole is withdrawn, leading to a function collapse. It could be the heart, lungs, circulatory system, brain, all or any of these and many more besides. As we still don't fully understand the workings of the human system the myriad reasons for its failure that we do know about are still short of their actual total number.

It could be a genetic weakness inherited from either parent or generated by their union, a microscopic invasion by virus or bacterium, fatal damage induced externally via accident or attack, illness brought about by the consumption of certain food or too much booze and smoke. Sheer bad luck. Age.

Death as a Way of Life

You are dead when your brain stops functioning. Normally it ceases to work because of a lack of oxygen caused by the heart stopping. The heart's function of feeding all the body's organs with oxygen is interrupted either because it becomes damaged or because the bodily functions that in their turn keep this powerful muscle going are themselves severely impaired or destroyed. All these things are very physical, specific and, at this basic level, not unduly complex.

However, this obvious and simplistic reasoning gives us insight only into that first question: 'How?' He died because: he had a heart attack; his kidneys failed; a brain tumour grew; a blood clot reached his lungs.

What it fails to address is the much greater mystery of 'Why?' or, more specifically, 'Why then?' At one given moment a person is alive, functioning, however weakly, and the next they are dead, gone. The switch has been thrown and whatever was the spark that caused the form to live is suddenly there no more. Something has departed, something tangible but without form, something real yet ethereal.

Life has a genuine presence that you can only really feel as it moves from a body. That is the sole time it shows itself, through its sudden absence. Though you cannot touch it, see it, or hear it, and while it is not truly tactile, life is nonetheless something one *can* feel, like electricity.

It is also true that one does not have to be physically close to sense the microsecond when it moves on. It is possible to perceive its passing at a considerable distance.

Whether the body physically moves or not, whether or not you can see a man's chest rise and fall as he struggles to breathe and then stops, whether or not you can see his eyes and the pupils dilating and then becoming fixed in that empty stare, the moment of the passing of life, the actual instant in which death replaces life is unmistakable.

Ask any widow who was by her husband's side at the end. Ask anyone who has witnessed a dreadful road accident and cradled the terribly injured in their last moments. Ask anyone who has been to war and seen front-line suffering.

Death, the moment when a person's lifeforce leaves them, is not signalled with a long exhalation of breath or a sudden limpness of posture. It is something else. The body may still be moving, may seem still to be breathing, to be alive. But suddenly, in a moment, before any death rattle or convulsion, something vital is missing, it's just not there. The spark has gone.

You can tell from 100 metres. Some people have felt it from a continent away.

From a clinical view, the moment of passing, the choice of the particular portion of time to die, is fascinating. At any one instant a patient is rarely noticeably any sicker or weaker than a second earlier. In the previous moment they were alive, only just, perhaps, but nevertheless able to function. Then, in the next, they are dead.

All I get is what is left. I can look at the evidence and establish what it was that caused the body to finally stop functioning. But I have absolutely no idea why it stopped functioning at that particular second, why one moment it could survive and the next it could not. Who turned off the switch?

As I say, the brain is the mainstay of life: while it functions you are a living being, whatever the state of the rest of you. The heart, lungs and kidneys can all stop functioning for a while and still the brain will continue. But if it quits, then everything else comes to a standstill.

When it stops, no matter if your body is marathon-man perfection itself, you're dead meat.

So what decides when the time is right to call it a day, the brain or the body?

Except in cataclysmic cases such as major physical damage, the time it takes to die can vary immensely in people with identical problems at apparently the same stage of their illness. One patient clings to life while another is gone at speed. A patient holds on and is neither worse nor better than he was hours earlier. But suddenly he dies, the effort stops. Why? What makes that final and irretrievable decision?

Does the mind have control over when it closes down? Can it pick its moment? Or is this a purely physical function; at a certain point of deterioration does the body simply send so many danger signals through the nervous system that it can no longer cope?

Normally the survival instinct is tremendously powerful, so what force of message would it need to receive to convince it to accept oblivion?

In the animal kingdom it is far from unusual for creatures to realize that they are going to die. When merely injured and still with a chance of recovery they will act in one manner. But when death is near, somehow they accept the calamity befalling them and have been observed to behave in very specific ways.

Among domestic animals, it is clear that cats like to die alone: they know when it's coming and prefer to make their peace in solitude, away from prying, gloating survivors. They know they are going to die and they prepare a place for the inevitable, going quietly, with no fuss.

Cause of Death

The cat's mind makes a conscious decision, as a consequence of its knowledge of impending doom, about where it will die. But how can it be so sure? Does it simply go to its final place and switch off? Is it possible they are so calculating and in control? Surely, if such matters were solely the province of the physiological, the cat would not be able to realize in advance that it was going to that big field in the sky and more moggies would be found stiff in the house rather than outside in a dark, peaceful cubbyhole, as they are, invariably.

In the wild, elephants are famous for their graveyards, their ancient instincts informing them clearly that death is going to happen soon. They live just long enough to make the journey.

That animals should seek a sombre place in which to die is not that remarkable. All thinking creatures have dignity and few like to suffer in public. What is fascinating is that once they have decided that they are going to die, they do. These animals don't have gloomy-faced doctors telling them their prognosis is bad: they simply read their own signs and know when their life is about to be over. Then, once in place, prepared and ready, something switches off their brain.

It is not unreasonable to consider that if a being is in pain the brain might be stimulated to read the signs, assess its body's damage and make a decision to close down, thus protecting itself from more agony in an already terminal situation. The physical entity might continue to cope but the mind chooses to grasp the inevitable a little early, to do its body a favour.

Equally, it would not necessarily be foolish to accept that the human brain, which still eclipses any bank of modern computers with its abilities, has the power to comprehend the notion of futility remotely, without referring the problem to the conscious mind.

Why should it not be able to assess the time when things are beyond hope and act accordingly, wasting no time on foolish bravado?

But then who is to say that the body as a whole is not the true controller of its final destiny? For eons tiny living things developed, improved and communicated without any brain at all. They responded accurately to changes in their environment, moving or operating in a direction or manner depending on what chemical, electrical, tactile or other stimulus each was receiving at any one time.

As evolution proceeded, that pure, natural reaction to a moment in life was superceded by what we now call instinct, where creatures responded defensively to several stimuli at once without really understanding why but knowing it was the smart move. Eventually, even instinct became obsolete as Thinking Man emerged to use his powers of reason, to use the advanced brain that allowed him to think before he acted. Surely it is reasonable to accept the possibility that all those old forms of communication are still within all of us, and the body can talk to itself without needing to go through the time-consuming and vexing process of thought.

Further, it would be foolish to rule out the intervention of a spiritual factor in the decision to die. The notion that the Grim Reaper, be he in the form of the Devil or the Archangel Gabriel, might have something to say about the matter is hardly new. This aspect, however, is certainly the one about which I have the least knowledge.

Like the mystery of life, the mystery of death is beyond us. But it does appear that each individual's time to die seems to be very specific to them and lacks the constancy that would allow us the opportunity to study the phenomenon properly and develop proof of a pattern that might allow us at least a glimmer of understanding.

Death, if possible more than life, is a singularly personal affair.

Life, of course, has been the subject of far more research than death and I had the privilege of being involved in one of the most important life breakthroughs of the twentieth century. The first 'test tube' baby, Louise Brown, was born at Oldham.

I was involved mostly at the beginning and, although I would not attempt to take credit for the astonishing result of the research, to this day I feel a bit like a distant uncle to the girl. Everyone who played any part at all in the process feels the same and we all follow her progress with interest.

Uniquely, Louise began life as a twinkle in the eye of two men.

Patrick Steptoe was the head of obstetrics at Oldham. While on holiday in France he called in at a hospital to see someone he knew and observed them using an instrument not then available in the UK. It was a laparoscope, a long thin tube with which one is able to pierce a tiny hole in the abdomen and then push through to view internal organs close up. Although it was quite widely used in France it had not crossed the English Channel, chiefly for one simple reason: the French, unlike the Germans and the Dutch, didn't then have their medical papers translated into English.

Steptoe knew straight away that this could have huge ramifications for his speciality of gynaecology and brought a laparoscope back with him. His explanation to Customs would have been interesting. 'It's a tube for getting into a lady's ovaries, officer.'

It allowed him to get close up to an ovary and identify problems there or in the uterus and was a fine diagnostic tool. Much later Steptoe learned that, by using another fine tube, he could extract an egg smaller than a pin head. To be able to do all this without the need for a major operation was a splendid breakthrough, the forerunner of keyhole surgery. (Mind you, if I personally were given the choice, I think I'd opt for a big scar. I'd prefer them to have plenty of room to work in if they were doing something tricky with my insides.)

Getting into the particular region of the body was one thing. But with so much going on in there, all squashed together, the field of view was insufficient to allow the surgeon to see properly, so the organs had to be separated. This we did by pumping two litres of carbon dioxide gas into the patient and swelling her up, so creating a larger abdominal cavity where it was easier to move around and locate what Patrick wanted to see.

Patient blower-upper was one of my tasks. Explain *that* to Customs.

Steptoe wrote a small book on the technique, which was well received, and he was invited to talk about his work.

Listening was Bob Edwards, a brilliant physiologist based in Cambridge, who realised the method would be very useful in the field he had chosen, fertilization.

Soon he was regularly travelling up to Oldham in his battered old VW Beetle and the pair began their laborious efforts. There was nowhere specifically where Bob could work so we let him have one half of a small room in the pathology lab.

Patrick removed the ova and Bob put them under the microscope to see how they responded to various situations. I was more than happy to carry out tests when they needed my help, not least because Bob was a charming man.

One of the first UK sperm banks was set up with the assistance of a number of suitable volunteers, young, healthy men who were, in fact, mostly medical students. The sperm was frozen with dry ice and tubes of cold seminal fluid were kept in containers that resembled small bombs. The sperm also needed monitoring to ensure that it stayed alive.

In 1969, the year man landed on the moon, the team managed the first-ever fertilization of a human egg in a lab, the first stage in achieving a test-tube baby.

There was an ethical storm about the process with accusations that doctors were trying to play God and had no right to interfere with the natural process of childbirth. The Catholic Church still frowns on the practice.

My own view is that it was perfectly legitimate medicine. Women who desperately want babies and cannot because of blocked or damaged fallopian tubes are suffering from a medical condition just as much as someone who is admitted to hospital for any illness or problem.

One way around this condition was to try to avoid having to use the fallopian tubes, to find another route for the sperm to take to get to the egg and then to do what it does naturally. They did this by introducing sperm and egg with the help of a micropipette and a Petri dish. I firmly believe that if a technique is developed that is clearly for the general human good then it should be allowed to prosper. In this case all they did was make it easier for nature to take its course.

In 1973 the team selected seventy-seven infertile women

to attempt the full job. Near the point they thought ovulation would occur, Patrick went to work with his laparoscope and brought out an egg that was then mixed with the husband's fresh sperm. Three of the seventy-seven became pregnant but none of the children survived to any late stage. One woman developed an ectopic pregnancy where the baby was developing outside the womb and Patrick had to remove it surgically.

In 1977 they again picked seventy-seven women, many from the first attempt, to try once more. They felt the first try had failed because of a hormonal problem and this time they used a different method to gauge ovulation times.

Each of the women who went to Dr Kershaw's Cottage Hospital, Royton, Oldham, which had become the test-tube baby clinic, was given a urine test and eleven were sent home immediately as unsuitable from a hormonal perspective.

Patrick got eggs from forty-four and from one of those he and Bob got their result. Mrs Lesley Brown, from Bristol, who was thirty-one years old and had been trying for a baby for twelve years, received an eight-cell embryo back into her womb on 12 November 1977.

Mrs Brown was the most cosseted mother-to-be I have ever seen and was given every test and aid the doctors knew. At four months it was clear that the pregnancy was progressing perfectly normally and Mrs Brown was sent home and told to take it easy.

Louise was delivered by Caesarean section at 11.47 p.m. on 25 July 1978. She was perfectly healthy and weighed 5 lbs 12 ozs.

The problems of establishing the precise time when eggs were ripe and ready for fertilization, retrieving them without damage, getting the sperm to take to an egg, incubating so the cells began to divide as they would in the womb and, finally, the delicate stage of implanting the new embryo back into its mother were soon overcome. The two men opened a private clinic in Cambridge to continue their pioneering work.

It is still a far from certain way of getting pregnant. But there are now thousands of children in the world who are living, breathing and laughing as a direct result of the work of Patrick and Bob.

Bob is still running the *in vitro* fertilization clinic at the time of writing this. But Patrick died of carcinoma of the pancreas in 1988 at the age of 74 on the day he should have gone to receive the CBE from the Queen at Buckingham Palace.

At his funeral a lot of people who didn't know him turned up. They were mostly under the age of ten.

6

The Police

The murder of a policeman is, thankfully, a rarity in this country. In fact, whatever the TV might suggest, the murder of a policeman in both Europe and the United States – even New York – is an unusual event.

One reason is that the police are all well trained to deal with situations where they may be at risk. They are trained in different ways because different forces in different countries need to be equipped to defend themselves in different ways.

Most countries' police forces are routinely armed with guns while ours are not. Illegally held firearms are much more prevalent in the UK than ever before and, as a direct consequence, the amount and range of weaponry available to the British police is greater than in earlier times. But we still do not arm our officers routinely even in the most difficult areas of our cities.

It is a situation I applaud.

Other countries claim, with justification, that the routine arming of their police officers helps them deal with difficult situations and has not led to more of their police being killed by gun-toting criminals. But that is not the point.

The point is that to arm officialdom encourages a gun culture throughout society. If it is legal for a policeman to carry a gun routinely it should be legal for an ordinary individual to carry a gun for self-protection. If most people carry guns then, naturally, a larger proportion of people with criminal tendencies will carry guns.

Usually, criminals do not open fire on the police for the simple expedient reason that they know that the police are generally better trained, better armed and better protected than they are. When faced with an armed police response, most people, unless utterly desperate or freaked out on booze or drugs, will, sensibly, throw down their arms, give up and try to con our jury-dependent court system. To do otherwise is tantamount to attempted suicide.

As discussed elsewhere in this book, guns make people dangerous. The more there are around, the greater the risk to you, me and the police. Anything that moves society closer to a friendly relationship with the gun should be avoided at all costs. For people here to get comfortable with the idea of patrol cops carrying pistols on their hips would leave me significantly unnerved.

The argument for British police routinely carrying such weapons is that they would have a much better chance of defending themselves against today's more violent and better-armed criminal. The argument has merit but it falls at an early fence: the cold statistics of recent history.

When you look at almost every occasion in Britain when a policeman or policewoman has been killed by a criminal's gun you will find that they had absolutely no chance of defending themselves. Nearly always the shot came unexpectedly in a relatively low-risk situation. If it had been apparent to the victims that they were entering a high-risk area, their training would have ensured they called for back-up before going into the incident. Being armed would neither have helped nor hindered, because it was simply not an issue.

In the States the police draw their weapons whenever a significant risk is perceived, when their high level of training tells them there is a potential problem. But again, most of their fallen comrades, if they died from the bullet, were shot when they least expected it.

The socio-criminal firearms problem from which the US and parts of Europe suffer is due partly to the fact that there the police expect to confront it more often. Fortunately, in the UK, even now, even the worst criminals do not carry firearms casually. The vast majority arm themselves for specific jobs and then hide the guns. To run the risk of being arrested as a known crook while carrying a firearm for absolutely no good reason would be an act of stupidity outrageous even by the standards of your average thick jailbird.

So, usually, but particularly in the United Kingdom (Ulster apart), unless you are looking for trouble and even if you are a patrol policeman, you have to be outrageously unfortunate to run into someone armed and actively homicidal. Of course, there is always some poor soul who runs out of luck.

Inspector Ray Codling was one such man.

He walked into the path of Anthony Hughes, a man as deranged and dangerous as any you might meet in your worst nightmare.

In 1960, at the age of thirteen, Hughes stole a bicycle and got his first criminal conviction. At fifteen he was sectioned under the Mental Health Act. Whatever punishment or help he received didn't work: as an adult he was jailed for ten years for a series of robberies, including one in which he fired a gun. On release, although he was an active homosexual, he raped an air hostess while posing as a policeman. The rape took place just two weeks after he was released. In total he spent fifteen years of his life in jail.

Later, obsessed with guns but prevented by his convictions from joining a gun club, Hughes made friends with members of a club in Diggle near Saddleworth, a smart village above Oldham. While there as a 'guest' he managed to steal a handgun, an Italian-made 9mm. Tanfoglio self-loading pistol that he secreted away for another day.

The weapon was next used two years later. Five days after that Hughes saved taxpayers the cost of a murder trial by pulling the trigger one final time to commit suicide at the age of forty-two.

He fired the gun's first 'angry' bullet in September 1989 when he aimed at a motorist during a wages snatch in Northenden, Manchester, not far from his home in Bagley, Wythenshawe. He missed.

Two days later Hughes walked into a bank in Hazel Grove, Stockport, and fired the handgun again, this time sending bullets into the ceiling before grabbing some cash, running out and jumping on a bus to escape. Yes, a bus. Just for the hell of it, he blew a hole through three of the seats on the top deck. Hughes was now totally out of control, crazed by what he perceived as the dirty tricks life had thrown at him. A near-friendless loser, a jailbird struggling with his sexuality, a victim, as he saw it, of society's myriad failings. His inner pain crushed him to the point where he broke. Free of any concerns for his own future he decided he wanted out. But first he wanted payback.

As the violent end became inevitable Hughes wrote letters to the five most important people in his life. He posted the messages through the office door of one of them, his Manchester-based solicitor, Kristina Harrison.

The other notes were to Hughes's stepfather, his gay lover, a relative in Birmingham and an elderly male friend in Preston. He wrote of his love for his stepfather, his boyfriend and his Rottweiler dog, Tyson.

In his letter to Miss Harrison Hughes wrote: 'I am extremely frightened. I don't know which way to turn. I have got myself into a fine mess this time and I am afraid it is over. I am going mad with tension. May God forgive me for my madness.'

With the police on his trail Hughes went on the run, sleeping rough and staying where he could while keeping moving on a Yamaha bike. When he parked up late one September night in 1989 at the Birch service station on the M62 motorway near Bury, Lancashire, he noticed two policemen in an unmarked car. It was not surprising, even at that time, two o'clock in the morning, to see officers at Birch as it is where the Greater Manchester Police motorway section has its HQ.

Inspector Codling, a forty-nine-year-old father of five, wound down his window and Hughes, apparently calm, leaned towards him to ask for directions to the cafeteria. The officer smiled reassuringly, pointed out the best route and watched as the biker headed off towards the service area's main building.

However, both policemen, professionally suspicious,

immediately turned their attention to where the leather-clad man had come from, stepped out of their patrol car and walked over to check out the rider's machine. They had no idea he was wanted for armed robbery nor that, later that day, he was due to appear before Bury Magistrates on five motoring charges. They never got the chance to have him checked out.

As they were looking at the Yamaha, Hughes silently and unexpectedly returned. Suddenly on his guard, the inspector's partner, Sergeant Jim Bowden, noticed in one glance that the crash-helmeted biker had a bone-handled knife in a sheath attached to his trouser belt and that his right hand was inside his short leather jacket.

Alert to the obvious danger of the knife the policeman reached forward to try to grab its handle. But it was already too late: there was no time to react, to defend himself against the imminent onslaught of mindless violence.

A sudden explosion made the sergeant stagger. He had no idea at the time but he had been fired upon. The bullet that would probably have claimed his life had hit the police-issue notebook in the right top pocket of his tunic and been deflected harmlessly away. The impact, however, threw him backwards.

Bowden watched in dismay as Hughes's gun hand swung away from him and the barrel was levelled at his partner. A second shot rang out. His friend fell to the ground. Then, no more than a second or two into this desperate horror, he saw the gun muzzle spit flame for a third time, this time into the back of his fallen comrade's head.

Sergeant Bowden, a forty-five-year-old father of three,

ran for his life, shots cracking out behind him. They all missed. A few moments later, when the firing had stopped, he instinctively – but not wisely – went back to try to help his stricken friend whom he could see lying face down, 'inert', as the officer put it. He tried to pick up Inspector Codling's nightstick and, looking around desperately, spotted the killer.

Hughes was crouching down by his motorcycle. As the sergeant spotted him, Hughes fired once more, this time more accurately. The bullet tore through the policeman's left leg but, despite the searing pain, Bowden found the strength to stagger 200 yards to the petrol station to call for help. The gunman could have easily caught him but, probably now in a state of panic himself, chose not to follow up on his semi-disabled target. Instead, he left the scene on his bike.

Sergeant Bowden lost six pints of blood in total but survived and was eventually to return to work. For Inspector Codling it was much too late.

I heard the news of the officer's death on the early-morning radio and was surprised not to have been called out earlier. Still, they had a policeman witness to the incident who could confirm the identity of the victim and the details of what had happened, so my findings were perhaps not paramount. It was eventually twelve hours after he died that I was able to begin the post-mortem at Oldham public mortuary on the body of Ray Codling. Coincidentally, it was at about that time that his killer was taking his own life.

The inspector was six feet two inches tall, well built and weighed a fit thirteen stones two pounds. The back of his head showed an entry wound, nine millimetres in diameter, two inches above and one inch to the back of the right ear. The left eye orbit had been destroyed by the exit wound.

There was a second entry wound on the outer side of the left forearm, again nine millimetres in diameter and this time seven inches below the shoulder with an exit wound on the inside of the arm and severely comminuted fractures of the left humerus. The bullet had passed clean through the arm, smashing the bone in its passage.

Another entry wound was visible on the left side of the chest and an exit wound, 1.5 centimetres in diameter and surrounded by bruising, was visible five inches below the right shoulder. The second and third wounds had been caused by the same bullet.

The scalp was bruised in the right parietal area, with fractures of the skull radiating from the entry wound in the right parietal bone, across the vault of the skull and into the frontal fossa. The bullet had passed diagonally across the base of the skull, causing haemorrhage over the surface of the brain and destruction of the left frontal lobe before entering the left orbit, destroying the left eye. While this would have been a certain-death injury, the officer was already dead or dying when it had been administered.

The lungs showed penetrating wounds on both upper lobes, caused by the bullet that had entered the left side of the chest between the second and third ribs. There was an exit wound between the second and third ribs on the right side. The trajectory of the bullet was exactly horizontal, fired at a man standing up and with his left side towards his assailant, perhaps beginning to turn away from or even to turn towards his killer. He might have been beginning to raise his arm defensively but, really, he had no chance.

The heart was normal but the pericardial sac contained blood and the pericardium showed penetrating wounds. Crucially, the front of the ascending aorta had been severely lacerated. This would have been instantaneously fatal.

In the hours after the shooting, Hughes who had been educated at RC schools, tried to find a Catholic priest, presumably to be his confessor. Fifty miles away in Kendray, near Barnsley, South Yorkshire, he approached David Walsh, the headmaster of a Roman Catholic junior school and asked where he could find the local priest, Fr Maurice Keenan.

Aware of events in Manchester, wary of the man's demeanour, his suspicions roused by the sight of the motorbike Hughes pushed into a garage at the side of the church, and knowing Fr Keenan was away at a funeral, Mr Walsh raised the alarm. A small squad of armed police surrounded the area and evacuated 114 children from the school. The officers waited outside the garage and Hughes would have known they were there.

He could have chosen to go out Butch-and-Sundance-style in a welter of blood and bullets. But he didn't. Instead, alone, without attempting a dialogue, still weighed down by the burden of sins unrelieved by a man of God and the sacrament of Confession, Hughes put the pistol to his head and pulled the trigger.

The bullet passed straight through his brain and he died instantly. It then exited from his skull, blasted through the garage door and embedded itself in a tree. The waiting police heard a crack and saw leaves fall from the tree. They waited thirty-five minutes before carefully opening the door and peering inside.

Hughes was lying on his left side on an old settee with his feet towards the door. The weapon was still in his hand, ready for firing with a further thirteen rounds in its magazine.

Hughes died much as he lived: alone, angry, armed, dangerous and somewhat pathetic.

When PC John Egerton, a strapping young man of twenty, went to arrest Arthur Edge, it should have been a straightforward matter. John was six feet three and well built with it. Edge was burly but unfit and tending towards fat.

The thirty-six-year-old petty thief with a string of convictions behind him was far from bright and had difficulty holding down a job. Bearing in mind that he liked expensive cars, this was a drawback.

For a while Edge worked for Dynamic Plastics, not far from his home in Farnworth, Bolton, but he was fired for skiving off during the evening shift. He had been unemployed for a year when he chose to return to the Dynamics factory for illegal purposes.

It was hardly the crime of the century. He clambered over the wall with a plastic container to syphon petrol from a car parked in the compound to use in his own. Typically, he was spotted by a patrol policeman, PC David O'Brien, who radioed for back-up.

John Egerton arrived quickly in a Panda car and, taking charge of the situation like the good copper he was, he told his colleague: 'You go that way, I'll go this.'

Both officers had their radios set for 'talk-through' so they could hear each other's conversations with the central control room. O'Brien was on the other side of the building when he heard control trying to raise John. No reply came over the air.

O'Brien walked around to the other side in pitch darkness, making his way carefully, listening for trouble. Suddenly his foot touched something soft. It was John, already beyond help.

The then Chief Constable of Greater Manchester Police, James (later, Sir James) Anderton, described his young, fallen officer as 'every mother's son'.

At three a.m. on the morning of Thursday, 11 March 1982, before his mother would have grasped fully the enormity of what had happened, before many of PC Egerton's friends and even some of his family knew of the tragedy and could begin to grieve, I began my work.

I first saw John fully clothed in police uniform at the Bolton and District General Hospital mortuary. It was clear immediately that he had suffered a number of injuries.

There were small abrasions on the right side of the forehead and right cheek and a deep laceration, half an inch long, on the right cheek, extending down to the bone. There were further abrasions on the nose, slight bruising of the right upper lip and a small bruise on the right side of the chin.

The trunk showed three lacerations of a jagged nature, also about half an inch long. The first was on the left side of the chest and had entered the chest cavity. The second was lower and to the left side and had penetrated deeply into the muscles of the abdomen. The last was at the same height as the second but to the front right of the abdomen; it had penetrated the abdominal cavity but missed the organs.

There were abrasions on the front of the right knee, the left ankle and the back of the right hand.

The heart was normal in size and shape but the pericardial sac contained a blood clot and there was a puncture wound at the apex. The myocardium showed a laceration at the apex of the heart with an exit wound on the posterior wall of the left ventricle that had penetrated the internal chamber of the left ventricle. There was a blood clot on the left side of the chest caused by the wound that had entered the chest cavity between the fifth and sixth ribs, cutting the costal cartilage of the sixth rib two inches from the midline of the body.

PC Egerton had suffered four stab wounds. The first three, to his cheek, his side and his stomach, would not have caused his death. The fourth, however, went straight through his heart, travelling upwards and inwards and penetrating the main chamber. Death would have occurred within seconds.

On the afternoon of the same day I was shown a kitchen knife with a six-inch blade that was half an inch wide at its widest point and had a single cutting edge. I assured the police this would have been capable of causing the injuries I found.

Edge was arrested before his victim was cold. He lived a few doors down, so close, in fact, that reporters interviewed his mother as they knocked on neighbours' doors to try to find witnesses to quote.

Ironically, unaware of her son's involvement in the killing, she complained to the journalists that, despite her complaints to the police, the area suffered badly at the hands of burglars.

Edge confessed to the police but then retracted his

statement and pleaded not guilty at his trial. It took the jury at Liverpool Crown Court just seventy minutes to find him guilty and he got life, with a recommendation that he should serve at least fifteen years.

Mr Justice Farquharson told him: 'Your brutality was matched only by the officer's own bravery and determination.'

John Egerton had caught the thief in the act and had detained him without too much trouble by putting him in an arm hold. Edge, in breach of three suspended sentences and terrified of returning to prison, pulled out the knife with his free hand and struck out ferociously. The blows would have come in quick succession, in which order it was impossible to tell, but the stabbing was over within seconds. Edge's victim didn't even have time to scream.

By way of worthless justification, the killer later told police: 'He just wouldn't let go.' John Egerton was that kind of policeman.

At PC Egerton's funeral the Chief Constable used the officer's own words as his epitaph. Two years previously, when the young man had filled out his application form to become a police officer, he had expressed his reasons for wanting to join the service in three simple sentences. Mr Anderton quoted them without further comment: there was no need, they spoke for themselves.

The teenage would-be constable wrote: 'I think it will be interesting, something I can take a pride in. I think it will be something I can do well and enjoy. I know also that I will be doing something useful and worthwhile.'

It was a fitting epitaph for that kind of policeman.

* * *

Another officer whose courageous decision not to let go in the course of his duty cost him his life was PC Ray Davenport.

He spotted a stolen car in Liverpool city centre with two young men in the front and three girls in the back. They had all been out for the night and had stolen a car, as was their habit, to get them home to the Old Swan area of the city.

At the wheel was Jeffrey Jaycock, nineteen. At his side was twenty-one-year-old Mark Kelly. Jaycock, who had drunk about six pints of beer during the evening, stalled the car that had earlier been reported stolen.

PC Davenport spotted them, realized it was a wanted vehicle and took his opportunity. There was no real risk, they were kids on a night out and this was only a stolen car, nothing serious. He reached in through the driver's window, as he had done on a number of previous occasions, to take the keys from the ignition.

An instant before he could get there Jaycock managed to get the engine started, slammed it into gear and sped off down the road. PC Davenport, thirty-five years old and the father of a teenage daughter, clung on.

Witnesses told of how sparks flew from the policeman's boots as the vehicle shot 200 yards down the road, careering from side to side.

Jaycock tried to push the officer back out of the window and Kelly leaned over to take the wheel from the passenger seat. The car slewed into a bus shelter and the officer took the full force.

A tough man, Davenport survived for two hours but died in hospital. I saw him at 6.20 a.m. at the Royal Liverpool Hospital.

There were two bands of bruising on the right side of the trunk, each about two inches wide and separated from each other by three inches. Drainage tubes, from the efforts of the doctors, were present on both sides of the chest. There were a number of abrasions, including a small one on the right middle finger. The digit also had a piece of glass at its base. More pieces of glass were in the constable's hair. Hair was found clamped in the palm of his left hand. He would have hung on to anything he could.

Internally, the scalp showed small abrasions in the front and occipital areas but the brain was healthy.

There were multiple rib fractures of the left lower rib cage with separation of the fragments. Ribs six to twelve inclusive were fractured in their posterior angles. On the right side there were more fractures of ribs at the costal margins but these were consistent with attempts at resuscitation.

On the left side ribs one to six were fractured at the mid angle and the deep muscles of the chest showed extensive bruising. There were sub-endocardial haemorrhages in the wall of the left ventricle.

The trachea and bronchi contained some blood. The lungs had a crush injury of the left lower lobe and crush injuries and lacerations of the right lower lobe. Blood was present in each pleural cavity. There was extensive blood in the peritoneal cavity and the liver had lacerations to the right lobe. The spleen, pancreas and thyroid were all healthy but there was a haemorrhage into the right adrenal. The left adrenal was healthy. There was bruising around the right kidney.

All told, the injuries were consistent with a heavy

violent blow to the right side of the trunk causing injuries to the lungs and liver. Hitting a bus shelter at more than twenty-five miles per hour would have done it.

Evidence of precisely who was doing what in the car was unclear, with each of the two defendants blaming the other, partially at least, for the crash. Their lawyers insisted they were 'overwhelmed with grief' for what had happened to Ray Davenport.

The jury accepted their pleas of not guilty to murder. Both were jailed for nine years for manslaughter.

PC Davenport's widow was not swayed by the lawyers' rhetoric and spoke vehemently after the case for the return of the death penalty.

She has an arguable point.

While Anthony Hughes was certainly certifiable, Arthur Edge was educationally sub-normal and the two Liverpool joyriders argued successfully they did not intend to kill PC Davenport, Clifford Lees had no valid excuse whatsoever.

Unemployed, Lees spent his time poaching in the woods around Chorley, Lancashire, close to the farmhouse where motorway patrolman Ian Woodward lived with his wife and two children.

Both as a policeman and as a good neighbour Ian, thirty-three, had been asked by local farmers to watch out for poachers, who had been making their lives a misery.

In late February 1987, he was walking near his home, off duty and in civilian clothes, when he came across Lees, twenty-four, who lived in nearby Clayton le Woods and was carrying a shotgun.

The policeman, used to life on the farm, would not

have been dismayed to see the weapon. It was a normal country situation. He identified himself and asked Lees to hand over the gun.

Lees refused. The details of the conversation between the two men will never be known but one thing is for sure: the policeman decided to back off. The other man had a gun and PC Woodward was a sensible man. He was out of uniform, acting only as a private concerned individual. The uniform, while offering no real protection at all, is often perceived as a useful tool in such circumstances, providing authority, control, and a measure of stability.

Ian turned his back and began to walk away. He would have been aware of the risk but probably not considered it high. Shotguns were commonplace around here. People used them to shoot small game, not policemen, not people dressed in civvies who had bumped into poachers.

It was at 3.35 p.m. on Wednesday, 25 February that I was taken by a senior detective to a field next to Chorley Sewage Works and was shown the body of a man lying face upwards on the ground. He was fully clothed and there were obvious wounds to his chest and neck. Rigor mortis had not set in and the body temperature was thirty-four degrees Centigrade. He had not been dead that long.

The body was removed to the mortuary at the Royal Preston Hospital and I carried out my examination. The subject was five feet, nine inches tall.

On the front of the neck, just above the sternal notch, was a ragged hole half an inch in diameter. Just below this and to the left was a slit wound, also half an inch long. The right shoulder showed another slit wound, again half an inch long, associated with bruising over the chest.

On the left side of the chest were two circular wounds that passed inwards and upwards to enter at the first and second ribs.

The back showed three circular wounds, each about half an inch in diameter on the right side of the chest, all within a tight three-inch radius.

Internally, tissues on the right side of the neck showed severe bruising, the lungs showed penetrating wounds in the right and left upper lobes and around the root of the lungs. The pleural cavities contained blood clots and blood on each side. There was a fracture of the fourth rib on the right side and bruising in the right fifth interspace where a metal shot was found. A gunshot wound had gone through the right scapula.

Subcutanial haemorrhages were present on the wall of the left ventricle of the heart, which was otherwise healthy, and there was bruising of the outer lining of the aorta.

X-ray examinations identified a further shot between the third and sixth thoracic vertebrae where damage to the spinal cord had occurred and a further shot was removed from the right upper arm.

The victim had received two distinct groups of injuries. The first, to the front of the chest, had passed upwards on the left side towards the right shoulder with injury to the lungs, tissues around the shoulder and the neck and penetration into the right upper arm.

The second group was to the right side of the back, damaging the right shoulder blade, the spinal cord and the right lung.

Either group could have caused death but the back

injuries were more severe and potentially more lethal. The policeman had died from massive haemorrhage caused by shotgun wounds.

The trial at Preston Crown Court heard that Lees first shot Ian Woodward in the back and then, as his victim screamed in agony, he calmly reloaded his weapon, looked at his victim's face, and shot him a second time through the chest.

Lees then went home, told his girlfriend what had happened and explained his murderous actions with the phrase: 'I didn't like his attitude. He didn't ask for the gun nicely.'

Lees, a rifle-club member, skilled with shotguns, pleaded guilty to murder. Two psychiatrists tried but were unable to find him insane.

Aware of what he was doing, aware of the consequences, Lees had shot the policeman twice, once while he lay helpless and in agony on the ground in front of him. Lees was sentenced to life imprisonment.

None of the deaths of these four officers could have been foreseen. Each went into what would normally have been a routine situation and died as a consequence. I cannot see, in the circumstances, how being armed with a firearm would have assisted any of them.

Codling was shot without warning, Egerton stabbed similarly, Davenport killed in a stolen-car dispute and Woodward while off duty confronting a poacher. None of these were armed-response situations.

The policemen, brave as they were, would have died in those circumstances however they were armed and whatever they did. Sadly, tragically, like being struck by cancer, it was their time.

Occasionally in life, the roof falls in. Most times there is the chance of getting the tile man out and rebuilding. Once in a while, though, it is a write-off.

Such was the case for a police constable in Cumbria in February 1978.

I had been called to a death in Barrow-in-Furness and was accompanied to Fife Street in the town by a detective chief inspector. I can only assume that he, personally, had not actually been to the scene of the death because the assurances he was giving me were almost by way of apology. 'Sorry to bring you all the way up here, I'm sure it's going to be nothing to worry about. As you know, we have to cover every eventuality.' He was convinced the deceased had met his death by an unfortunate accident.

Anticipating a quick departure and return down the M6 I walked into the house and was somewhat surprised to be shown the body of an adult male lying face upwards at the top of the stairs.

I stood back to try to take in the whole situation and attempted not to cast an eye in the direction of the optimistic DCI. 'That's blood on the walls', I told him, as gently as I could. 'And that's a piece of skull! And that over there is a piece of the dead man's brain.' He got the picture.

We had a very violent murder scene. The blood was scattered around the walls close to the dead man's head, and small pieces of brain tissue were near his left foot. Two pieces of skull were near the right foot.

Jack Groombridge Dodd, aged sixty-four, had been the victim of a dreadful, frenzied attack. At four p.m. at the public mortuary in Barrow I began the examination.

Dodd was five feet, three inches tall and there were lacerations to the left side of his forehead. One was one inch long, above the left eyebrow and surrounded by bruising, the second was triangular and near the top of the head on the left side. To the right of the forehead there was an abrasion three-quarters of an inch in diameter, and at the back of the head on the left side were three ragged lacerations between three-quarters of an inch and two inches long. They were consistent with having been caused by a blunt instrument.

In the cranial cavity there was extensive bruising on the back of the scalp with extensive fractures of the skull involving the left occipital bone which was severely comminuted with extensions to the left parietal bone. In the midline, near to the front was a separate depressed fracture of the vault. The brain showed surface haemorrhage with extensive lacerations of the left occipital lobe and the left lobe of the cerebellum.

Dodd's heart and lungs were beginning to show the signs of a hard life and old age. But he had died from a cerebral haemorrhage caused by a fracture of the skull, itself caused by multiple blows to the head, at least five.

Unusually, I stayed for the detectives' conference after the post-mortem. During this they run through the evidence they have so far and decide how to proceed with the rest of the inquiry. A number of uniformed officers who had been involved at the start were also present on this occasion.

As questions and answers unfolded, one of the uniformed men started to go white. He was clearly unwell and staggered slightly. Being a doctor, you notice these things. Being a forensic pathologist in a room full of cops I knew that the best course of action was to do nothing until requested to assist. The request never came and I went home.

The policeman went home, too. But the following morning he approached his boss and told him that he believed one of the suspects in the murder case should be his own son.

Mr Dodd had been in bed at his home when sixteen-year-old Martin Barnes, his neighbour in Fife Street and the son of the police constable, broke in. The youth, who had been drinking, wandered around the house and, too noisy ever to be a decent burglar, let his footfalls be heard as he walked upstairs.

Mr Dodd came out of his bedroom, glanced at the boy he knew and was hit with a claw hammer. He went down straightaway. Follow-up blows were probably unnecessary but they were administered anyway. I told the court the victim's skull resembled a jigsaw puzzle.

The teenager admitted most things. He had broken into his neighbour's house to steal but had been caught red-handed.

Barnes told his father's colleagues at Barrow police station: 'When I got upstairs Dodd must have heard me. When he came out I hit him. I went into his room and couldn't find anything, then I walked down to Greengate Bridge and threw the hammer over the wall. I never meant to go in and hurt him. I'm sorry I caused any bother.'

Barnes pleaded guilty to manslaughter but, armed with my evidence of multiple blows, the prosecutor, David Waddington, QC, later to be an undistinguished Home Secretary, argued that the boy had returned to the prostrate and helpless old man and had hit him again to silence any possibility of identification.

It took the jury at Preston Crown Court just an hour to

find the teenager guilty of murder. He was sentenced to be detained at Her Majesty's Pleasure.

He will probably be out by now.

While I have little sympathy for such a violent young man, I hope his father has recovered. Rarely have I seen an individual become sickly so suddenly.

7

Mad or Bad?

Absolute evil, however it is defined, is rare. In peacetime it appears in one place perhaps no more than once in a decade or so. War, of course, gives all those people on the edge of evil the opportunity to exploit the situation.

On those occasions when it does appear we tend to try to find an excuse for it. We don't excuse the actions, of course, but we often try to excuse the perpetrator. His or her behaviour is so horrendous, so far outside what most people consider to be reasonable behaviour, that we try to place them outside our own social grouping.

In short, there is a tendency to accept quickly that anyone who can do such terrible things must be mad.

The initial plea of Peter Sutcliffe, the Yorkshire Ripper, that he was 'not guilty to murder but guilty to manslaughter on the grounds of diminished responsibility' was accepted by the prosecution. It was only the refusal of the trial judge at the Old Bailey to accept, without the judgement of a jury, that Sutcliffe was insane that finally allowed him to be convicted of the cold-blooded murder of more than a dozen young women.

While, realistically, the outcome would not have been too different, the 'guilty' verdicts for the charges of murder were nevertheless highly significant. Sutcliffe's wish to plead guilty to serial manslaughter would have produced as significant a number of life sentences as he actually received for being found guilty of the same number of murders. Whether he is bonkers or as sane as the judge, he is clearly a lifetime menace and must be locked up until he is too old, weak or ill to harm anyone.

However, the judge's – and ultimately the jury's – decisions provided us with a sheaf of verdicts of guilty to murder: premeditated, brutal slayings of young women that were not in any way mitigated by Sutcliffe's state of mind. They provided us, the watching, fearful and traumatized public, with a wanton, savage killer. Sutcliffe will always be considered a foul, deadly murderer, not – as his shrewd defence lawyers wanted to portray – a twisted unfortunate who was as much a victim of his tortured mind as those poor girls he slaughtered.

The Ripper, we can be satisfied, did what he did because he wanted to, knowing it was wrong and fully comprehending the consequences. He did it because it was evil, not because he was insane. That was the decision of the court. The verdict allowed us all to hate him freely, without the diluting redundancy of also having to pity his desperate soul.

Pure, unsullied hate, well directed and entirely defensible despite its obvious vengefulness, can provide good therapy for an individual or a society. One might ponder whether the judge's decision was based solely on law and precedent or whether wider influences insisted that Sutcliffe had to be pilloried for other reasons. In truth, I have no idea, so let's stick with the point.

Before Sutcliffe came Moors murderer Ian Brady, a man now clearly insane and doubtless destined to die in a secure psychiatric institution. However, at his trial in the mid-

1960s his defence was not that he was a paranoid schizo-phrenic. His defence was that he didn't do it.

After Sutcliffe in the middle 1970s, came another violent inadequate who might have become as notorious as the other two but was stopped before he really got into his stride.

When Trevor Joseph Hardy finally came to court after killing three young girls the jury was set a tricky task by the defence: tell us, they asked, is our client mad or bad?

Like Brady, Hardy had a close woman confidante who was aware of the atrocities he was committing. Unlike Myra Hindley, it was never proved that Sheilagh Farrow ever played any active part in Hardy's murders. However she did supply alibis and harboured him in the full knowledge of what he was and what he had done.

After Hardy's arrest Farrow did a deal with the police to save her own skin, providing damning evidence against her savage lover in return for immunity from prosecution for herself.

To this day the families of Hardy's victims are striving to have Farrow prosecuted.

To this day – assuming she is still alive – there is little doubt that Farrow is much more concerned about Hardy getting out than about anything the judiciary might do to her.

At Hardy's trial an eminent psychiatrist suggested Farrow's 'ex' was a 'very dangerous psychopath' who would remain a significant danger to the general public for a considerable length of time. That doctor was called by the defence.

Hardy was thirty-one-years old when he came to trial in 1977 charged with the murders of three girls over a fifteenth-month period between New Year's Eve 1974 and March 1976.

I had professional contact with only one of his victims. She was the first to be killed but the last to be found.

Janet Lesley Stewart met her death at the tender age of fifteen for no better reason than that she was in the wrong place at the wrong time. The misfortune that took her young, innocent life could be compared to being struck by lightning. Her last thoughts, while no doubt dominated by terror, would have been filled with absolute confusion. She was killed by a man she did not know for a reason she could never have guessed.

Hardy's penchant for criminality first came to the attention of the authorities when he was just eight years old and was caught housebreaking. An archetypal school bully, he preferred to use his fists rather than use what was a higher-than-average IQ to solve arguments. With each victory came a punishment and with each punishment the chip on his shoulder grew ever greater.

By the age of fifteen he had absconded fourteen times from approved schools and had pleaded guilty at Manchester Crown Court to burglary and larceny, asking for twenty-one similar offences, all committed over a two-month period, to be taken into consideration. Despite the offender's youth the judge took the exceptional step of sending the boy to adult prison.

Prophetically, the young Hardy was told: 'In your case the public needs to be protected and the only conceivable course open to this court in these circumstances is to send you to prison where you will be securely held.'

By the time he was arrested for murder Hardy had accumulated a criminal record of 147 separate offences. They, of course, were only the ones for which he had been caught.

The young Hardy became a well-known thug in North Manchester. He was just five feet, seven inches tall and quite slim. But his build disguised surprising strength and a hard-as-nails spirit that made him, in the words of his contemporaries, 'a hell of a scrapper, impossible to put down in a fight'.

In private, though, this tough guy was unusually close to his mother and, despite making claims to the contrary, had relatively few normal relationships with girlfriends. Occasionally, he enjoyed dressing up in women's clothes.

One odd friendship of Hardy's was with Beverley Driver whom he met when she was an adolescent, ten years his junior. He started hanging about with her and her teenage friends, becoming a sort of 'leader of the pack' not because of any inner dynamism but simply because of his age.

Hardy claimed Beverley and he were lovers but she always denied the suggestion, insisting they only ever kissed and cuddled. Her account has always seemed the more plausible.

In 1972 Hardy was jailed for five years for wounding a man called Stanley O'Brien, an offence for which he always vehemently insisted he had been framed. In prison he festered over the 'injustice' and vowed vengeance on his accuser.

While incarcerated he received news from Beverley that doubled his fury. On advice from her parents, she wrote telling him that she could no longer have anything to do with him and was breaking off their friendship. She also let slip that she had a new boyfriend more her own age. That put her alongside O'Brien on Hardy's hit list.

He told friends inside he had two reasons to live: to kill them both.

In November 1974, just a month before Hardy was to vent his murderous fury on a helpless teenager, he was released from prison and went to live with his mother at her home in Brentnor Road, New Moston, Manchester.

To his staggering disbelief he discovered that his primary target, O'Brien, had died while he, Hardy, had been serving his time. His hatred for Beverley increased accordingly.

The following New Year's Eve, drunk as usual, Hardy left the house armed with a kitchen knife and started to roam the streets. Later he claimed his intention was not random violence; he was, he always insisted, looking for Beverley.

On Ten Acre Lane he saw a girl get out of a car and heard her speak cheerfully to the driver. It was Lesley on her way to meet her boyfriend at the nearby Phoenix Hotel and join pals for a night out. She was laughing loudly and easily.

The driver said: 'Goodnight Lesley' and drove away. Hardy was eventually to suggest he mistook the word 'Lesley' for 'Beverley'.

One feels that the true likelihood is that whichever young girl he came across that evening would have met a similar awful fate.

Lesley, pretty, dark-haired, a former Rose Queen at her local church, was probably surprised by the man who approached her out of the gloom but it is unlikely she was immediately intimidated or frightened. In 1974 most women were safe on the streets and, after all, this was New Year's Eve, a night when strangers often spoke to each other.

She didn't get a chance to say much. By Hardy's account,

just four single-syllable words phrased in an obvious question.

Hardy said: 'Do you remember me, Beverley?' and the bemused youngster replied: 'What do you want?'

Lesley never got her answer. Hardy lashed out with his powerful arms, muscles used to street fighting, and punched the girl in the face. She went straight down and he kicked her as she lay on the ground. Then, when she was helpless, when he must have seen her face clearly, when he must have known this was the face of innocence, the face of one who had never done anything to harm or anger him, he produced the knife.

A single strike, he said, to the throat. He remembers blood pouring out of the side of her neck which suggests he severed either the carotid artery or vein.

Despite the fact that, clearly, Lesley was dying before his eyes, Hardy did nothing to help. He just stared, motionless, as she choked, gasping for breath and grabbing uselessly at the terrible wound. She would have been unconscious in less than one minute and effectively dead in three.

'I just stared and watched,' the killer later confessed to police. Then, in a sentence phenomenal in its utter selfishness, he added: 'I didn't give a damn after what I'd been through.'

Hardy dragged Lesley's body into a hollow, covered it with grass and then calmly walked home to watch Andy Stewart's Hogmanay Show on TV with his mum.

Later that night he climbed out of bed and returned to the scene of the murder. He carried the corpse further into undergrowth not far from Moston Brook High School and buried Lesley in a secluded shallow grave.

Over the next few months Hardy returned to the body

with knives and an axe and removed several pieces. Sometimes he used his bare hands. It would have been possible to dismember a body without instruments after only a few weeks if rapid decomposition had taken place, which was the case here in wet ground. The bones would separate almost as easily as they do on a cooked chicken.

Having said that, it would have been a particularly gruesome and unpleasant task: the sight, smell and feel of rotting flesh is disgusting, as is the sound it makes when it is pulled away from the bones it covers. Hardy said he went back to prevent identification of the corpse but one could easily argue he actually returned more for some very strange form of gratification.

When the detective in charge of the case, Charles Horan, called me to the scene at 5.30 a.m. on a fair morning in September 1976 the area was quiet and we had plenty of room to move without too many people getting interested.

I was shown a piece of bone jutting out of the soil where the police had been digging and I stood by as the careful exhumation took place. The body was little more than a skeleton with insubstantial pieces of skin, cartilage and muscle attached. A trench was dug in front of the area of the grave and the team worked backwards, uncovering what was there an inch at a time in an attempt to disturb as little as possible of the remains. They were bones only, but lying in the configuration of a body.

It was a very shallow grave, so much so that it was surprising it had not been discovered earlier by that man walking his dog who always seems to instigate these inquiries.

The body was lying on its back, the legs outstretched and the arms by its side. It had, in undertaker parlance, been 'laid out'. The extremities, that is the head, the hands and feet were all missing. Also not present, perhaps oddly, was the right femur, or thigh bone.

Pathologically there was little to go on but, usefully, it was clear that the growing end of the bones of the upper arms had not fused. This indicated that the dead woman – for clearly it was the corpse of a female – was under twenty years old. Beyond that age the skeletal structure alters to a point that in normal activity makes no significant difference but accounts for why girl gymnasts are at their flexible best in their youth.

On that day the search provided me with a left clavicle (collar bone), a left scapula (shoulder blade), left humerus (upper arm from shoulder to elbow), left radius (the thicker and shorter of the two bones of the forearm), left ulna (the inner bone of the forearm), the complete bones of the left hand, twenty-two ribs, twelve vertebrae, one sacrum (a triangular-shaped bone at the base of the spine), the left pelvic bone, the left femur (thigh bone), left tibia (inner bone of the lower leg from the knee to the ankle) and fibula (the longer bone on the outside of the lower leg) and the right tibia and fibula. The length of the femur was seventeen and a half inches, which established the victim's maximum height at five feet, ten inches.

Five days later I was shown at the Manchester mortuary a number of other bones that had been uncovered later at the site. These were two vertebrae, a right clavicle, one rib, a right fibula and one ankle bone. The age and development were consistent with the bones found previously and were likely in the circumstances, to be from the same individual. All told, we had about half of the girl's skeleton.

Further searches of the area failed to provide us with any

more of the victim's body. While we could not reasonably expect to find the remains of small, separated hand and finger bones, we were disappointed not to find the head. Clearly it had been disposed of with some effort elsewhere.

Hardy claimed he had decapitated the corpse and thrown the head into a nearby lake that had subsequently been filled in.

His attempts to disguise her identity were wholly successful. There was not enough left of the body to indicate any more than that this was a young woman who had died within the previous five years.

That these were the mortal remains of Janet Lesley Stewart, from Harpurhey, Manchester, aged fifteen on her last birthday, who had vanished on the first day of 1975 was impossible for me to say. We only had Hardy's testimony for it but, for once, no one doubted him in the slightest.

Shortly after Hardy became a killer, he met a woman ten years his senior, the aforementioned divorcee, Sheilagh Farrow, and soon they set up home together in a flat in Smedley Road, Newton Heath. On one occasion when he returned to Lesley's body he removed her ring and watch. After polishing them up he gave them to his new girlfriend as a birthday present.

In July 1975, six months after the first murder, Hardy was to strike again in a chillingly similar – but even more violent – fashion.

He didn't know seventeen-year-old Wanda Skala, a part-time barmaid at the Lightbowne Hotel, any more than he knew Lesley Stewart. But, once more, brutal lightning was to strike. It was just Wanda's misfortune to meet Hardy in a bad mood.

Drunk again and broke as usual, he had just had a row

with his lover. He says he initially only intended to 'mug' the teenager, robbing her of her purse, as he was out of cash.

The results of a post-mortem carried out by my Home Office colleague Dr R. Cyril Woodcock showed starkly that this was no simple mugging gone wrong: this was savagery at its most extreme.

Wanda had been waylaid as she made her way home from the Lightbowne after a late-night staff party. Her head had been shattered by repeated blows from a large stone that was found nearby, heavily bloodstained. Her own socks were tied around her throat. She had been kicked powerfully and repeatedly in the genital area. Most shocking of all, the nipple on her right breast had been bitten off.

In a statement Hardy said: The murder started as a robbery but the girl struggled. I hit her on the jaw. She collapsed and I carried her round behind some boards and left her. Then I went back, tried to strangle the girl, couldn't, so picked up a brick and hit her in the face four times.

'I had been reading a book from the library on murders and had read about the Heath case and decided to make it look like a sex attack.' (Heath was a notorious murderer in the 1940s who killed two girls and sexually mutilated their bodies.)

Hardy was an immediate early suspect in the Wanda Skala killing but Farrow provided him with a cast-iron alibi. On the night in question, she told detectives, he had never left her side.

Subsequently Hardy was to try to implicate Farrow in the killing, claiming he had murdered Wanda because his girlfriend was present during the mugging and he feared that the teenager might recognize her. Farrow always denied this but accepted that she had cleaned Hardy's bloodstained clothes.

If we are to be generous and accept her account of events then Farrow was not a party to the actual killing. But she readily provided an escape route for a man she could reasonably accept was guilty of a heinous crime.

She knew Hardy had the opportunity to kill the girl, she knew he returned home with his clothing spattered in blood that was not his own and she knew he had a tendency towards violence.

If the blood was from a straightforward street fight, why should she lie? Why does any woman lie to protect a violent man? It is something that happens all the time and something I cannot comprehend.

Hardy's younger brother, Colin, had much better sense than Hardy's besotted mistress and attempted to put an end to the slaughter. He had for years been afraid of his big brother, having seen his short temper and easy way with violence. But he had put up with it, as brothers, sisters, wives, mothers and girlfriends often do.

However, shortly after Wanda's death, while the community was still traumatized by the emerging horrific details, and while the two men were drinking in a local pub, Trevor Joseph leaned conspiratorially to Colin and admitted: 'It was me.'

It was not an apology, nor a confession; it was a boast.

The pair walked back to the flat nearby where Colin lived with his wife, both sobering up with each step. The younger man was shocked and sickened by what he knew was the truth of what he had been told and the older one was beginning to realize the enormous danger in which he had placed himself with such a frank admission.

When he was sufficiently clear-headed, Trevor Joseph quickly resorted to his favourite weapon of control – violence. As the two men reached the flat and stepped inside he attacked his brother without warning, beating him senseless with his fists and feet before turning to stroll back into the night.

Five minutes later, while Colin's appalled wife was trying to tend to her injured husband, still prone at the bottom of the stairs and with blood congealing on his face, the door opened and Hardy stood over her.

Apparently calm, he walked past the moaning mess of his brother and coldly but civilly asked the terrified woman if she would make him beans on toast. She complied without question. This was a man with all the social graces and charm of a carnivorous beast and she wisely took no chances. Fed, he stood up and left, walking again past the still semi-conscious form of his brother.

Colin recovered from his mauling but his fear now knew no bounds. He genuinely believed he and his wife could be his brother's next murder victims. The beating, clearly, was to prevent him speaking about what he knew. But what if Trevor decided that was insufficient insurance? What if Trevor came back to make certain of Colin's silence?

The terrified man went to the police to shop his homicidal brother. As it turned out, it wasn't that great a move.

Detectives arrested Trevor Joseph Hardy and brought him in for questioning. However, a second-hand confession from a member of the family who might have an axe to grind is not the most compelling of evidence. It was no more than a start in producing a case to answer in court.

Nevertheless, there was plenty for them to look at. The teeth marks, for instance. Hardy was a reasonable suspect for a number of reasons but he would never crack under the pressure of questioning. He'd been through that sort of thing too many times.

But the killer *had* left his bite print on his victim. The marks on the edges of Wanda's severed nipple were like a fingerprint to a forensic odontologist.

This was something that occurred to Hardy and he spoke of it to Farrow. She dutifully smuggled a file into her boyfriend's cell and, during hours alone, he spent his time with the hard metal in his mouth, scraping the rough, iron-hard edges against his teeth, meticulously and as silently as he could – bearing in mind the pain – filing them down to points.

When the bite check was made it was clear to the dental experts that Hardy had been working on the shape of his teeth but the best they could conclude was that the marks were 'not inconsistent' with his own bite shape. That lack of conclusiveness married to the alibi provided by Sheilagh Farrow, allowed him to be set free pending further inquiries. And to kill again.

In March 1976 Hardy attacked a girl in a pub toilet. He squeezed her throat so hard she bit through her own tongue. Disturbed before he could finish the job, he fled and lived rough for a few days, knowing he was being sought.

The girl was very fortunate. Hardy was later to say: 'I throated her. That usually works.'

Three days after that attack he claimed his third young victim.

Sharon Mosoph, seventeen, from Failsworth, near Oldham, had enjoyed a staff party at the Pack Horse Hotel,

Bolton and was returning home by bus. She got to Piccadilly, Manchester shortly before one a.m. and then caught a second bus to Broadway within walking distance of home.

As she passed Marlborough Mill, where she worked, she noticed someone in the shadows. Hardy, drunk and penniless again, was trying to break into the factory.

Like the other victims, Sharon never had a hope. The moment Hardy saw her he lunged and hit her with the screwdriver he had been using to force the door. She screamed, struggled and tried to run away but he caught her by her dress, swung her towards him and stabbed her in the stomach.

Another young girl was in his way, in his face, causing him problems. Her death became his entire ambition. Though she was already dreadfully injured, Hardy decided to inflict much more damage. His feet were somehow in the wrong place to give him maximum power so he gave himself better leverage by bracing his foot against a wall to allow him to choke her until she ceased to breathe or move.

Sharon was found floating in a canal with her tights around her neck. Her left nipple had been bitten off.

Peculiarly, Hardy later claimed that he committed the mutilation to put police off the scent, clearly a foolish notion. He always refused to admit that he gained any sexual pleasure from his abominable actions.

It was not long after returning to the flat in Stockport that he now shared with Farrow that Hardy realized he had left behind significant clues.

In something of a mirror image of his first murder he returned once more to the canal, located the body and dived in. Using a rivet, he slashed across Sharon's mutilated breast sixty-four times to try to erase the imprint of his teeth from the wound where her nipple had been.

My colleague Dr R. Cyril Woodcock was called out to this case. It was one of the first investigations ever to use a video camera at a crime scene. Chief Superintendent Tom Butcher, a well-known character in the police, was organizing the whole affair. It was, understandably a fairly harrowing business because of the state of the body and he was not in the mood to be messed with. He spotted someone, a member of the public, leaning out of a building, trying to get a view of what was happening and Butcher screamed at him to, shall we say 'go away'. It added a certain something to the video-footage soundtrack, which, as evidence, could not be tampered with or altered.

The similarity between Wanda's and Sharon's killings took the police back to Hardy and he was charged with both murders, although the police felt their evidence was far from complete.

Farrow, who had previously cold-bloodedly supplied the alibi, cracked and told them everything. When Hardy discovered this betrayal he told everyone who would listen that he would hound Farrow and would exact his revenge.

She was told that if she gave evidence she would have full immunity from prosecution for involvement in any of Hardy's activities, an offer she gratefully accepted. Twenty years on, the families of the victims are still trying to reverse that decision.

In August 1976, while on remand for the two killings, Hardy asked prison staff if he could speak to a detective about something important. He provided a remarkable confession. Out of the blue he admitted killing Wanda and Sharon and added a third death to his sheet, that of Lesley

Stewart, a teenage girl who had been reported missing and whose whereabouts were still a mystery.

Hardy had been routinely questioned about Lesley, but his denials of any knowledge had to be accepted by the police at the time as there was no evidence to suggest he had been involved in any way with what had happened to her. There had been, after all, no body, no confirmation of her death.

It was after Hardy's confession that I got involved when I got a telephone call from Chief Superintendent Charles Horan, the head of Manchester CID.

One might have thought that the fact Hardy had been able to take us all to the site of a third murder and then help in the location of severed limbs would have been in itself evidence enough for a successful prosecution. The lawyers, however, wanted it ironclad. They were as afraid of this man as any other sane individual and were desperate to secure a life sentence.

The forensic evidence was good, but not compelling. The confession was wonderful but could always be retracted.

Mrs Farrow was used as the belt to go with the braces. The thought of Hardy going free on some technicality or on the whim of a jury was unthinkable. He was a serial killer with a potential murderous future ahead of him; she was just a lowlife who had been reeled in to his scenario. No one really thought that, alone, without her bruiser mate, she was capable of being significantly dangerous. His conviction was considered to be worth any compromise, no matter how distasteful. Farrow was small fry. She got her immunity.

At the beginning of the trial Hardy pleaded not guilty to all three murders, despite his confession. Three days into the evidence he changed his plea to: 'Not guilty to murder but guilty to manslaughter on the grounds of diminished responsibility.' In other words, he claimed the defence of madness.

Hardy's counsel spent the rest of the trial attempting to persuade the twelve jurors that Hardy was suffering from a medical condition that made him terribly dangerous – but not through any fault of his own. He was ill, desperately so. He needed help, not punishment.

The prosecution, for their part, took the view that Hardy was simply a nasty piece of work who killed because he felt like it. He killed because he was angry, and he killed indiscriminately. By coincidence or not, his victims were all innocent young girls. He committed these acts, they argued, because he was evil, not because he was ill.

And the jury agreed. Hardy, they decided, was bad, not mad.

They took the view that evil and insanity do not have to be bedfellows, that the sanest of men can commit the worst brutalities. Killing does not have to be the act of the deranged.

It is a principle with which I completely agree, even though it is a woefully depressing sentiment.

Hardy was found guilty on three counts of murder. A life sentence was mandatory. As this book is published he is still in maximum security and has passed his fiftieth birthday.

Recently a rumour circulated that he had been released on parole. As soon as they heard this, senior detectives made frantic attempts to check with the Home Office that he was still securely incarcerated and were relieved to discover that the rumour was nonsense. Hardy was still locked up.

Had they heard the same rumour, even greater fear and

then relief would have been felt by two of his ex-girlfriends, his younger brother, and most of those who ever came into contact with Trevor Joseph Hardy.

The newspapers called him 'The Beast of the Night'. Rarely has any man had so terrifyingly appropriate a title.

8

To Have or Have Not

In 1993, after between 30,000 and 70,000 Bosnian women had been made pregnant by wartime rapists, the Pope wrote to the Archbishop of Sarajevo, Vinko Puljik, and asked him to pass on a message from Rome.

The leader of the Catholic Church, arguably the most influential man on earth, urged the women: 'Do not abort. Your children are not responsible for the ignoble violence you have undergone. Accept the enemy and make him the flesh of your own flesh.'

The following day a prestigious Italian newspaper ran an article supporting the Pontiff's view and portrayed the issue at stake not as one of rape but one of illegitimacy. It praised the Catholic faith for giving its blessing to women who were having the illegitimate babies of the invading soldiers.

In the same year Cardinal Basil Hulme, the then leader of the Catholic Church in the United Kingdom, backed the Pope's condemnation of abortion as an 'unspeakable crime'.

In America abortion clinics have been targeted by violent protests and five people who support abortion have been murdered by anti-abortion fanatics. The argument that the fanatics make is that the American law of 'justifiable homicide' applied. This law states that one is justified in using force, lethal if necessary, against an aggressor to save a life.

In January 1997 two bombs exploded at a family

151

planning clinic in Atlanta, Georgia. Intelligence reports suggested that American anti-abortion 'terrorists' were planning to cross the Atlantic and disrupt the British General Election.

I wonder if David Steel, the now knighted former leader of the Liberal Party, knew what he was letting us in for when he negotiated the Abortion Bill in 1967.

Abortion has a remarkable history over a much longer period than people might imagine. It was first made illegal in Britain in the early 1800s. Naturally, as a consequence, backstreet abortions became big business but in 1861 another law that made it illegal to 'procure a miscarriage' was passed. Anyone who supplied or used 'poison or another noxious thing or other means' to induce an abortion was liable to a term of life imprisonment.

Despite this the illegal trade continued to flourish, as did the sale of 'women's remedies' that caused a severe irritation of the stomach and bowel and, occasionally, a miscarriage. DIY abortions were also popular with desperate women prepared to use crochet hooks, knitting needles, lead solutions, soap, hot baths, gin, and heavy blows to the back and abdomen. They were even ready to take an out-and-out kicking.

In 1936 the Abortion Law Reform Association was formed, aiming to lift restrictions on doctors to allow them to offer safe, legal abortions. Two years later a gynaecologist, who performed an abortion on a fourteen-year-old rape victim, was acquitted by a jury on the grounds that he had acted to preserve her life. That was the first time that the health of the mother had been accepted in law as grounds for an abortion.

The outbreak of the Second World War interrupted any

further reforms. But in the 1960s the case of the thalidomide children and the birth of other deformed babies
brought the questions back to the fore. The thalidomide
drug, it is argued, didn't actually cause the loss of babies'
limbs, but it was an abortion suppressor that prevented
nature taking its course by bringing to an end an imperfect
pregnancy. Consequently the drug allowed some births to
take place that might not otherwise have progressed to full
term. This counterweight to the earlier argument simply
inflamed the debate once more.

It was in 1966 that Mr Steel decided to sponsor the
Abortion Law Reform Bill in the teeth of opposition from
many colleagues in the House of Commons, religious
groups and sections of the medical profession. It was passed
in 1967 and became law in April 1968, legalizing abortion
under specific criteria in England, Scotland and Wales, but
not the Isle of Man, Northern Ireland, nor the Channel
Islands. (The Manx legislature finally passed the law
twenty-seven years later.)

In 1990 the Human Fertilization and Embryology Act
was passed, bringing down the upper time limit for most
abortions from twenty-eight weeks to twenty-four.

Whatever your stance on abortion, everyone must
applaud the one great success of the Act which was to
reduce drastically the number of backstreet abortions. No
one knows how many were being done but estimates vary
between 40,000 and 200,000 a year before 1967.
According to the British Medical Association between
thirty and fifty women died of the effects of illegal abortions each year.

In the twenty years after 1969 the number of abortions
each year more than trebled from 54,819 to 186,912, but,

of course, those were legal operations only. By 1990 single women accounted for 67 per cent of all abortions.

However, in the good old days when the worst thing that could happen to you after having sex was to become pregnant, single women accounted for probably 95 per cent of backstreet or DIY abortions. I recall two quite vividly, both, as it happens, occurring shortly after the new laws were in place. The first woman, unusually, was married.

Sandra Elaine Beardow, aged twenty-two, was admitted to the Oldham and District General Hospital in a collapsed condition on 4 April 1969, and died shortly afterwards. It was suspected she had undergone an attempted abortion involving the injection of an antiseptic solution. It turned out that the abortionist had used Dettol.

Sandra and her hairdresser husband had one child, two years old, and did not want another. They either did not ask or were turned down for a 'contraceptive' abortion and went instead to a house in Banff Road, Longsight, Manchester, the home of sixty-year-old Jean Hammett, a backstreet abortionist of many years' standing.

Sandra's heart was normal in size and shape but the pericardial sac contained blood-stained fluid and the lungs were oedematous (swollen). The liver was soft as was the spleen, which was also slightly enlarged. The pancreas, thyroid and adrenals were healthy but the kidneys were moderately enlarged and showed mottling consistent with septicaemia.

The uterus was enlarged, corresponding to a two or three months' pregnancy, the placenta was practically separated and the uterine cavity contained a dead foetus of two to three months' gestation. Frothy, blood-stained fluid was also present and seeping from the vagina.

Swabs were taken from the vagina, uterus, chest tissues,

the heart and the spleen. In each case bacteriology tests showed the presence of Clostridium welchii, a deadly bacterium. Sandra had probably picked it up from the instruments used or something in the room where the procedure was carried out. She died from blood poisoning.

The introduction by syringe of the Dettol would have achieved its primary objective which was to separate the placenta from the uterus, thus shutting off the flow of blood to the foetus and causing it to die. But that can leave an open wound ripe for infection. Many abortionists believed the disinfectant would prevent such an occurrence. No doubt it sometimes did help, but not always, and not in this case.

Hammett was jailed for two years. Passing sentence, Mr Justice Crighton told her: 'The real evil of that which you did is shown by the result. The ghastly danger in which young women who have abortions of this sort with insufficiently cleaned instruments find themselves is seldom realized.'

Three years later I performed an autopsy on Joan Percival who was only twenty years old when her married boyfriend kindly attempted to give her an abortion in the back of his Ford Corsair.

I drove to Tarporley War Memorial Hospital, Cheshire, where I was first shown her body on a trolley in the operating theatre. Then I viewed the bronze-coloured car that had in the back seat a pump, a plastic syringe, a plastic tube and wet towels.

At 5.30 p.m. on 19 February 1972, I began the examination and noticed a soapy solution was present in the vagina. The skull and meninges were healthy but the surface veins showed some air bubbles. The brain was oedematous but otherwise healthy. The heart was normal in size and shape but there were subendocardial haemorrhages in the wall of the left ventricle. The right ventricle contained blood and air bubbles. The inferior vena cava contained some drops of soapy solution and the lungs were congested.

The cervix showed small abrasions around the cervical canal where there was a plug of mucus. In the uterus, which was enlarged, was a male foetus of approximately sixteen or seventeen weeks' gestation. The placenta was separated around the edge.

There was no sign of septicaemia in this case. Joan had died from an air-and-soap embolism. Both had entered the bloodstream and moved around the body until they reached the heart, blocked a blood vessel and caused a build-up of pressure until it ruptured.

The boyfriend, Robin Luckhurst, was jailed for a year by a judge at Chester Crown Court after pleading guilty to manslaughter.

Joan had initially been friendly with Luckhurst's wife and became pregnant after she (Joan) and Luckhurst began an affair. She saw a doctor but, frightened to face the truth, delayed going back for the results. When she eventually had her condition confirmed she attempted suicide before being referred to a gynaecologist. The court heard that he told her the pregnancy could not be terminated because of the delay.

She and Luckhurst tried several DIY methods to carry out an abortion, all without success. Then, as a last resort, they drove to a secluded lovers' lane near the village of Little Budworth and he used his pumping kit in an attempt to administer the solution.

Clearly Luckhurst got it wrong and the young lady died

in pain. While the insertion of the tubes should have caused no significant discomfort, the separation of the placenta would probably have been extremely unpleasant and Joan was clearly, according to his evidence, very distressed before she died.

Luckhurst told police he became alarmed when Joan started crying and her complexion changed colour, so he immediately drove her to Tarporley Hospital. Sadly, she was dead when he got there. 'I didn't know the seriousness of what I was doing,' he said. ' I didn't realize the danger.'

If he'd had half an ounce of sense he *should* have realized the danger. The termination of a pregnancy is a major procedure. If it was easy you wouldn't need doctors to perform it.

The moral situation is a minefield. While modern thinking states correctly that a woman should have the right to choose how she lives her life, there is a real question over how her rights override those of a developing foetus.

This modern woman, with all her choices before her, decides to have sex. Fine, but she should accept the responsibility of any consequences of her libidinous association. The product of her union has no such choice and should be given every natural opportunity to achieve its potential to survive to be one of God's creations.

To many that is a compelling argument even without the spiritual overtones. The religious argument is the unequivocal statement that, once the sperm and ovum have merged, life at that moment exists and cannot be taken by anyone other than God – for any reason. But the fact that the foetus at that stage cannot exist outside its host, the mother, allows a number of interpretations of the situation.

Cause of Death

I was deeply involved in the test-tube baby *in vitro* fertilization project that successfully examined and overcame some of the difficulties of birth. During experiments it was necessary to use human embryos: the work could not have succeeded otherwise. The towering achievement of that research is that a large number of people today who could never have had children together in a 'natural' sense are now parents. I am proud of that work and I believe that the experiments on the embryos were worthwhile and utterly justifiable.

That statement will alienate me from the many who believe any invasion of God's natural process is a violation. Certainly the 'pro-life' lobby will not take to me kindly.

But there is so much they stand for with which I am steadfastly in agreement. Abortion as a routine form of contraception is wrong and life is sacred. The group of cells in the womb will, given a chance, become a fully formed human being – and the opportunity for that development should be given every chance. No one could argue against that basic truth.

My difficulty lies with the use of absolutes. Many things were written in stone eons ago because no one envisaged them ever becoming capable of being less than utterly solid. They were certainties, morals, Commandments; they were medical facts.

During the past fifty years our global awareness has increased at a rate beyond the imaginings of our recent ancestors. The men who put Man on the moon in 1969 could not begin to understand the workings of today's simplest digital watch. Medical science, medical knowledge, medical boundaries of achievement are all expanding at a quadratic rate. The routine procedure of today was only theoretically possible a short time ago, while the possible of now would then have been regarded as a near-miracle.

Before long medicine may be able to guarantee to protect the life of every conceived foetus to the point of birth by non-natural means. Is that an act of God? I wonder if the pro-life lobby would approve.

In this matter I only ask the questions, for I genuinely have no answers. And I suspect there are no answers that will satisfy everyone.

While people concentrate their efforts so often on the beginning of life, there is occasionally a remarkable concentration of the mind at the end of it that causes all kinds of problems.

Back in 1970 I was asked to examine Alice Ashworth, a lady who had survived seventy-seven years and resided at Moore Street, Rochdale. I was asked to visit her home and found her lying in bed in the front downstairs room. She was dead, I could tell straight away.

We took her to the mortuary and measured her at just five feet in height. She was partially clothed and in a state of extreme mummification. There were no obvious external abnormalities.

The skull was intact, showing no evidence of fracture, the meninges were healthy but the brain was partially liquefied. The blood vessels showed severe arteriosclerosis. She had severe emphysema and the right lung was thickened at the base and was adhering to the right side of the chest.

There was a small crack fracture of the neck of the left femur. I was satisfied that the elderly lady had died from pneumonia following that fracture. I was also satisfied that she had been dead for about six months.

Cause of Death

Alice Ashworth's husband had been looking after her in their small terraced home. It appeared from what he said that she had suffered a fall and he had put her to bed. She had died and either he hadn't realized she was dead or he could not accept it. The latter is the more likely. It is not that unusual among the elderly who have spent more than half a century together and can't imagine being parted.

Somewhat disconcerting, however, was the widower's statement that he had noticed Alice was a bit cold so, during the previous six months, on a regular basis, he fed her hot soup.

9

The Moss

In Victorian times, perhaps the smartest residential area in Manchester was an exclusive neighbourhood less than two miles from the centre, along the southward route out of the city. Houses there were large and grand, the homes of well-to-do business folk continuing to prosper from the fresh opportunities and progress brought about by the Industrial Revolution whose heart beat strongly in this part of England which, after all, was its birthplace.

Typically, these houses were brick-built and double-fronted, with at least six bedrooms and two reception rooms. The large basements would be occupied by a small staff of perhaps three people; a butler, a cook-cum-house-keeper and a maid to attend to the lady of the house. On Sundays, all the families would dress appropriately, go to church, and then spend time at leisure, the men mixing business with pleasure, checking on their friendly competitors' latest gadgets or schemes.

At the turn of the century it was both comfortable and fashionable to live here in the adjacent districts of Whalley Range and Moss Side.

Nearby, in order to service the burgeoning factories, hundreds of small terraced houses were thrown up. Each new row of small, two-up two-down homes steadily extended the boundaries of this briskly growing smoky metropolis that sprawled outwards in every direction.

Entrepreneurs were, in the main, successful, so much so that some of the money made actually filtered down to the workers, though obviously not too much. The factory types still knew their place and it seemed only proper that working-class folk should doff their caps and curtsy to their betters. Things, of course, changed.

During the first half of the twentieth century two World Wars took their toll on the workforce. The revolution that had provided a whole new way of life first peaked and then slumped towards obsolescence, choked by the very innovation it had inspired. The great mills and factories whose production and pollution had characterized the landscape for so long became quiet, empty hulks, the carcasses of once-proud industrial mammoths, extinct, their roles superseded by more modern requirements and more productive, inventive methods and means.

Before many more years passed the neglect that inevitably troops behind unemployment like a mangy dog afflicted the weary buildings. The terraces, built honestly but for an earlier, less demanding age, fell into disrepair and degenerated into uninhabitable slums.

After World War Two, improvements in transport and the arrival of less salubrious neighbours caused the wealthy to move out to leafy suburbs further removed from the grimy city. As a consequence, the smart Victorian houses were sold to sharp developers who spotted a growing niche market and made fat profits turning the homes into rented flats.

Rightly, the authorities decided that human beings should not have to live in slum squalor and bulldozed all the old outside-toilet cold-water-only terraces. Unfortunately, what was built in their stead was in many ways somewhat worse.

Whilst the fabric of the old homes had become truly dreadful, the people who inhabited them had, nevertheless, managed to hold on to an enlivening and protective sense of community. Their lives might have been extremely difficult, but they knew that they were in it together.

These were people who still spoke proudly of the Dunkirk Spirit. Even though these Mancunians had never seen the sea and would have most impolitely refused an invitation to board a rowing boat on Heaton Park lake, they were of the same game stock as those courageous mariners who had evacuated nearly 340,000 British troops from a Northern French seaport in 1940, despite the relentless attacks of German forces. These were people, who had been through wars together, folk who had protected each other against a common enemy, who had been drawn together in that cause, who had survived not least through that togetherness. The post-war period was still a time when people could leave their doors open while they popped around the corner and not have to worry about what they'd find when they returned.

However, all this was ignored and the leather-taut community fabric was shredded, its people split up and housed variously elsewhere. The community itself was wiped out, its strength replaced with fragility. Its power to control itself, indeed to police itself, drained away like the slurry of the building sites that quickly sat atop the sad remains of its old homes.

The people were spread across the city, thrust into new-build New Towns, all strangers to each other. These strangers suddenly found themselves in a new world, surrounded by faces they did not recognize. The spirit that had carried neighbours through the darkest of dark times was too diluted ever to regain control. Bad housing and unemployment had been tough enough to cope with, but the ruination of the once-solid community was probably the worst single mistake of the many made during these rapidly changing times.

This was a period of social mutation that was to take us all down a path to an entirely different way of life, one based on values and aspirations alien in many respects to those that had previously been considered important.

History shows that the Common Man had certainly been abused by those with the power to do so. But throughout his trials he had retained both his pride and his honour. In pursuit of vengeance for this unjust deprivation, New Man sacrificed too much of his honour and replaced it with most of the Seven Deadly Sins. Rage, envy and greed, the three most volcanic, appeared first, with gluttony and sloth following close behind this ugly transformation. Pride was the only solid thing many people had to hold on to but even this later showed its sinful side. The seventh Sin, lust, which also predominated, caused no more problems than it had before. For it to have done so would, of course, have been as impossible then as it is now.

The answer to the housing problem was at first thought to be high-rise flats. By building tall you could put roofs over the heads of a lot of people while using up only a small area of precious ground. But this policy led to isolation and depression. People had been used to passing time with other people by moving about outside their homes and indulging in gossip and laughter. There were many benefits to that kind of entertainment, the most important being that, like a lot of the best things in life, it was free.

But in these impersonal blocks of flats the families had no obvious access to their new neighbours, nothing to draw them out of their hutches to mingle and form a new community. Across the old yard wall they would chat and share. But in lifts they stood silently, staring at the flashing light counting down the floors, and held tightly on to their shopping.

Further, many of the flats were outrageously badly built and the thin walls, floors and ceilings offered little protection from the pollution of cold, damp and noise. Although this was a time several years before it was customary for families to stay in all night watching TV, these folk abandoned their chattering and changed their lifestyles, becoming 'flat hermits', their ears open to the radio, hearing about the outside world but, for the first time, less prepared to enter it.

Suddenly the outside was threatening.

Realizing their error, the planners responded by making another mistake. They invented deck-access accommodation. This was supposed to be terraced housing in the sky whereby homes were set next to each other, each with their own Coronation Street-style front door but with one 'street' sitting immediately above the other, up to five storeys high.

Unfortunately, the buildings were so ugly and, either because of corruption or ineptitude, probably both, so appallingly built that people were asking to move out literally within weeks of being moved in. Almost beyond belief is that one such block, demolished to everyone's relief after twenty years, was based on the design of the magnificent Crescents in the city of Bath.

Finally, they put people back on the ground in tradi-
tional-type homes. But yet again, they made mistakes.
These new houses would probably have been the perfect
replacement for the slums the town planners had levelled
in the early 1960s if only they had been provided at that
time. There were yards to chat from, gardens to sit in,
gates and walls to gossip over. The homes had mod cons
and were, for the most part, solidly built. There were
walkways and small squares where people could pass time
together. This was a place designed for a community to
flourish.

But they had forgotten one vital thing. The community
had gone, been tossed to the four winds, and with it had
vanished that solid centre of collective preservation, that
ability of neighbours to act together and control the more
destructive elements in their midst. It was no longer 'all for
one and one for all'. It was 'all for me'.

This, together with a 'new wave' of selfishness, envy and
greed on the part of too many individuals, the inability of
socially blind or cowardly politicians to realize what was
happening and the consequent failure of the police to
address the situation sufficiently quickly, inflicted the next
blight to strike humanity in the inner cities: endemic criminality.

If ever a place was designed for the criminal it was the
new Moss Side. There were scores of places to hide and,
from each, at least four places to run. Walkways and little
squares led to a confusion of overpasses and underpasses
and the police, who had long since stopped using their feet
and taken to motorized transport had no chance of catching
the young muggers, burglars, thieves, and – new on the
block – the drug dealers who thrived there. Being a criminal

in this part of Manchester was very soon to become child's play in more ways than one.

And here there was a further problem that, in time, was to become probably the biggest: the question of race. Postwar Britain needed labour and invited in the people of the Commonwealth and other poorer countries to join us. As it happens, the Commonwealth and the poorer countries are primarily non-white. So a large number of coloured immigrants arrived on these shores, more than content to take unskilled jobs that provided a much-improved lifestyle to that which they could reasonably expect in the less developed towns back home.

For reasons that still baffle me, councils across Britain decided the best move was to keep these immigrants all in one area. In London, Brixton was one such place; in Bristol, St Paul's; in Liverpool, Toxteth; and in Manchester, Moss Side was chosen. I am not suggesting that black people did not live elsewhere as well, of course they did, but significant numbers were placed together. It seems that no one involved in devising this policy had ever heard of the American experience.

In the States they were already thirty years ahead of the UK in terms of racial difficulties at the time this was happening. But no one chose to take notice.

In this country, in the early 1960s, if you had put a significant number of French immigrants, visiting Poles, newly arrived Swedes, itinerant Australians or runaway Swiss in one place you would have noticed a gradual natural shift in that local society for the perfectly obvious reason that fresh cultural ideas would have been assimilated into the fabric of everyday living. That is not to say that any such changes would have been entirely trouble-free and without difficulty for, sadly, it appears that some problems are inevitable when cultures collide. But, in general, few casual observers would have noticed. Those driving through such areas wouldn't have spotted anything odd, those heading for the shops would have failed to see anything bizarre. Just a bunch of ordinary-looking Brits going about their business, apparently.

But put a few hundred Afro-Caribbeans on the street and things are different. Let's face it, they are black.

Now, humanity has always been tribal and warlike: that is how it survived to take over the planet. Even before it developed a modern brain and stood up straight it knew that there was safety in numbers, not only from the animals it hunted and that hunted it, but also from the other hominids who were the only genuine threat to it. Tribe fought tribe for territory until wisdom prevailed and humanity learned how to exercise restraint, to draw a line and keep a truce, to negotiate a mutually beneficial peace, to use its unique power of speech for its own good.

Blood, as we all know, has always been thicker than water. Man has always distrusted that with which he is not obviously bonded – indeed, as Cain taught Abel, even those who for family reasons *should* be close are often far from brotherly towards each other. Man's inhumanity to man is legendary and, sadly, is as malign and virulent today as it has ever been.

Man likes to have an enemy because he enjoys victory. Without an enemy, an opponent, it is impossible to demonstrate superiority. Armed with victory, he can display his supremacy to others and expects as a consequence to be held in higher esteem. This battle can take place anywhere, at any time, between any number of individuals and in many different forms, some harmless, others not so.

Battle is joined, for instance, in the workplace where one individual strives to achieve better results than someone else or be promoted faster. Attracting the prettiest girl in the room or simply winning an argument once more provides satisfaction from victory. This conflict and competition is everywhere and gives us parameters by which we can assess both our own performance and that of others.

To feel safer, because that conflict is everywhere, we tend to band together in groups. Some groups are very small, a husband and wife, for example, while others are larger, such as those of football supporters. At any party groups will develop, consisting of people who have things in common. Often they split up into sections based on sex, age or profession. Or race.

Two white men in a room full of black men will find each other as will two black men in a place packed with whites. It shouldn't be particularly surprising, it is simply that the natural, protective tribal need to bond pushes together individuals with things in common. It is the same with two young people in a room filled with the elderly, two women in a place full of blokes or two pathologists surrounded by paediatric psychologists.

Racism is the belief that one man is better than another simply because of racial origin. At that level it is a wonderfully silly concept that falls at the first fence. The place where you are born bears absolutely no relationship to the man you will become. The society into which you are born, the quality of your parents, the amount of opportunities you receive, your genetic make-up, your good fortune or lack of it, all these things matter. But all can vary to a near-infinite degree wherever you happen to be born.

Racism as we have come to know it actually has little to do with a genuine belief that a white man is better than a black or vice versa. It has to do with identifying an enemy. The black men most hated and feared by whites in America and more recently in South Africa have not been those whom the racist might reasonably consider were inferior to himself. Quite the reverse. They have been those who are demonstrably intelligent and powerful. Dr Martin Luther King, Malcolm X, Nelson Mandela, these men were feared not because they were lesser men but because they were hugely successful. The black man was not primarily an enemy because he was less than the white man, he was an enemy because he was readily identifiable as different, of a different clan. And you could see it at a glance.

In the 'civilized world', for want of a better expression but most notably in the New World, America, the black man was captured into slavery by the white man and subjugated until the inherent good in most of us saw the light and won the day. But the black man was now out of Africa and into Europe, America and the islands of the Caribbean, and realized – rightly – that he was still seen by probably the majority of whites as a former slave, a second-class citizen. He was angry and his sons were even angrier and this made them intimidating.

The white man bonded with his own kind and the now-free black man found life was almost as hard without his shackles as it had been before. Low incomes, bad housing and the code that insists that people of the same kind will bond together conspired to create the black ghetto. From New York to Chicago to Detroit to South Central Los

Angeles the American ghettos grew and the people inside them festered in poverty. They became very dangerous places to be, particularly if you were white. Whatever your politics, whatever your understanding and sympathy, whatever reason you had to be there, if you were white you were a target. Because you were different, no other reason.

It was a simple progression, an obvious conclusion. But we in Britain didn't see it coming.

Moss Side's black population grew throughout the 1960s and 1970s and racism flourished. If a black family moved into a street the house prices fell. This was because of the attitude of the white buyers, but it was the blacks who got the blame. It didn't matter whether they were a decent family or a set of hooligans, their very colour set them apart. These were not logical times.

In truth, many of the black families did not help themselves. While the Asians of India, Pakistan and China (via Hong Kong) integrated and profited from a powerful work ethic and close family ties, many Afro-Caribbeans were perceived as being lazy. It may have been a misunderstanding or it may have been an accurate assessment, I am not in a position to know, but it is certain that they were considered the least welcome of the various immigrant communities.

Work became harder for blacks to get with some companies 'blacklisting' certain areas. The post codes of Manchester 15 and Manchester 16 figured on several firm's lists. Across Britain certain areas with large Afro-Caribbean populations became notorious for crime and civil unrest and in 1981 there were riots in the black areas of several cities, including Manchester. The police station in Moss Side was under siege for two days and nights until the police came out with a mandate to hit anything that got in their way. Order was quickly restored but, in the eyes of the greater public, 'black' was now associated with 'riot'. Racism had another excuse.

It was after this orchestrated violence that politicians began to take the situation seriously and try to do something about the places that were starting to turn into ghettos. Black or white, it didn't matter, if you lived in one of these places you tended to be stuck there. This was the new exception to the old rule of it not mattering where you were born.

The second and third generations of black youngsters were kids with Manchester accents and black faces. Their heroes were black men on the television, beamed into their homes from New York, Chicago, Detroit and South Central Los Angeles. Their heroes were black men who got even.

It is not surprising, given all the circumstances, that street gangs should have been spawned in such a potent and unedifying mixture. Fortunately, our natural fear of guns has ensured that it is unlikely we will ever get to the hopeless state of many US cities and the number of young gangsters actively working the streets here is still very low. But they still manage to cause a major problem.

In the early 1990s in Los Angeles, there were two main gangs, the Crips and the Bloods. There were 30,000 Crips and 9,000 Bloods. Around that time many of them chose to move east and the vacuum they left behind was filled by Jamaican 'Yardie' gangs. Between them they are believed to have been responsible for spreading 'crack' cocaine across the entire North American continent.

At the same time the entire population of Moss Side was

only about 14,000, with about 6,000 being non-white. There were two main street gangs, the Gooch and the Doddington, both about thirty strong. They were mostly in their late teens or early twenties and some were connected to Yardies based in London and Kingston, Jamaica.

While criminal behaviour was taking place throughout the inner city it was in Moss Side that a great deal of the drug trafficking was carried out and it was these gangs that did it. The layout of the area allowed them to move freely and avoid capture. The dealer would take an order on his mobile phone and agree a contact point. A twelve-year-old lookout on a mountain bike would be able to spot any danger and warn the dealer. The drugs would be carried by a ten-year-old on another mountain bike because if he was stopped by the police nothing would happen to him due to his age. The deal would be done and the cash stashed until there was too much of it to be safe. The dealer would then walk into a BMW showroom and drive away in a 325i or nip into an estate agency and buy a small house for cash.

Profits were considerable by the standards the dealers set themselves but that was not the primary driving force. Status was much more important than wealth. These young men needed respect and would go to quite appalling lengths to achieve it.

I do not know how people so young can be prepared to become involved in such dreadful violence. But then, in times of war they are actively encouraged to kill and maim and usually make the grade. The Doddington and the Gooch had their own war but for such weak reasons that it did seem rather pathetic.

There are three types of violence in a drug culture: that

committed while under the influence, that committed to get money for drugs, and that committed by gang members against each other for whatever reason.

Although it is usually assumed that most inter-gang violence is associated with the protection of 'turf' this was not the case in Moss Side. Here, status was all and neither side would back down.

It took so little provocation for matters to end in death. On one occasion members of each faction fell out and punched one another. In any other walk of life that would have been the end of it. But no, neither side could let it end there: they would have lost face. Soon afterwards a car was stolen from outside a drinking den; then another fight and a Doddington man lost part of an ear; then a car was set alight and a gun discharged on Gooch territory. Thirty minutes after that an attack was staged on a Doddington pub and a man was macheted. Two weeks later a Gooch was stabbed; then the Doddington pub was attacked again, this time with a 9mm handgun being fired; then a Doddington was shot and a Gooch macheted; then two Gooches were set on fire by Doddingtons who poured petrol over them. Doddingtons were then fired upon and finally, inevitably, a Gooch man was hacked to death with a machete.

These individuals were fearless. They were not concerned about being arrested, about life in prison, about being injured or dying. They actually enjoyed the buzz they got from being shot at and loved the 'respect' that access to a gun and money provided for them. It was all that mattered. It gave them Pride.

Fear was the key to success and extreme violence was the method employed to guarantee that fear. One drug user from Birmingham was told the price had just gone up when he went to a house in Moss Side. He refused to pay and was shot in the face with a sawn-off shotgun. It wasn't necessary to kill him but it was done anyway. It increased the fear factor.

Guns were used regularly. But fortunately most of the ammunition the dealers could get their hands on was of poor quality so an unusual number of shooting victims survived the attacks. One man lived after a bullet passed straight through his head, ricochetting around his skull but missing any vital parts of his brain. That, while a miracle of one sort, was, as you can imagine, also a gift from the gods for the purveyors of racist gags.

Cars were regularly fired upon and later discovered abandoned with bullet holes in them. Official complaints were hardly ever made to police. Most gang members wore bulletproof vests as a matter of course and consequently assassinations had to be carried out at close range. Julian 'Turbo' Stewart was shot in the head by a man he thought was about to shake his hand.

A seventeen-year-old boy was hacked to death by a number of youngsters wielding machetes. He had more than twenty-five separate wounds. Another was chased into a local butcher's shop and blasted to death in front of shoppers. Amazingly no one died when a man stood on a table in a pub and sprayed the room with bullets from a MAC-10 machine gun. This was the stuff of video violence – but for real.

Even when they were arrested gang members continued to get away with it. They simply ensured that any potential witnesses were visited and warned in no uncertain fashion what would happen to them if they gave evidence. Several trials collapsed because of this tactic.

In 1993 a masked man walked into a takeaway food shop in Moss Side, singled out a tall black youngster and killed him with two blasts from a shotgun. The dead boy was called Benji Stanley. He was not known to police as a gang member and, although his size belied his age, he was just fourteen years old. His death led to a national outcry and a new initiative by Greater Manchester Police.

The police operated on two fronts. The first move was to try to salve old wounds between themselves and the wider community and to persuade the people on the estates that the police were a better option than the drug dealers. The next was to set up a special unit to target gun crime in the city.

It was known as VO15, run from Longsight police station, two miles from the Moss Side trouble spots. It was headed by an experienced Detective Chief Inspector called Kevin Haigh, a likeable man from Oldham whose outwardly gentle demeanour disguised a fierce determination to complete the task at hand. Within eighteen months his hand-picked team had enjoyed considerable success, playing a large part in imprisoning many of the leading players among the gangs and taking scores of weapons off the streets.

However, as one man fell another was ready to take his place and there was much skirmishing among the younger, wilder elements. Older heads, fed up with being shot at and weary from the fresh impetus of the police, called a Manchester-wide truce. Now disputes were solved by payment in cash rather than blood. If someone stepped out of line and revenge was required, the avenger would be paid from the gangs' collective funds. The payment was sufficiently respectful for 'face' to be saved and no further action to be required.

That worked for a while. But, inevitably, new people, mostly young and reckless, came to the fore and, while the Moss is certainly in better shape today, both socially and economically, than it has been for decades, it still has a long way to go to achieve its aims. The drug gangs are still very much part of the local fabric.

For a tiny minority the law of the gun remains the favoured method of settling disputes. These, still, are not arguments over drugs, turf, firearms, or any of the things most people would assume a gangster considers important. They are over trivia. A stolen bike, a mistaken glance or a throwaway remark can result in a call to the pathologist.

Sometimes, with unerring stupidity, people, convinced of their own power, set themselves up by attempting to 'tax' other gang members. This is a dangerous tactic expressly designed to achieve 'face' through fear and attrition. In the short term it can work if the violence or threat of violence is sufficiently extreme. Usually, though, the longer-term prognosis is fatal.

The Moss, as it is known, has been destroyed, rebuilt, used and abused by all kinds of people for close on fifty years. In recent times a small number of demotivated and extremely nasty young men, the waste products of a cruel and mean society, have given it a notorious reputation that cannot be denied. But it is good that this level of violence is still shocking to people in this country. The Moss has been and remains occasionally a relatively dangerous place, but it will never be in the same league as New York, Chicago, Detroit, or South Central Los Angeles.

Gang Culture Case Studies

As I have explained, most gang-related killings in inner-city Manchester were not directly connected to the control of drug runners' 'turf'. It could be a factor in the outbreak of much of the violence but business matters were usually settled sensibly.

The loss of turf was acceptable to most gangsters if they had sufficient reason to let it go. But if that move involved any loss of respect then matters could get out of hand. The loss of respect was utterly unacceptable in any shape or form.

For instance, if someone was prepared to give up turf for a price, then that was a business transaction. If someone who lost turf was later compensated by either the new area boss or, indeed, anyone else keen to keep the peace, that too was OK. Should anyone choose, for his own reasons, simply to abandon turf, not a problem.

It was the respect, not the turf, that counted. As in most walks of life, the workplace – in this case the street – was not the most important thing in the lives of young men. Their home lives, their relationships, their families were the most important things. They were more likely to have a loss of respect here than 'at work'.

Peter Walker, a gang boss in Hulme, was jailed for life at the age of twenty-one for the shotgun killing of another drug runner, Henderson Proverbs, aged twenty-five. Ludicrously, the murder followed a fight over a woman between two other men. Neither Walker nor Proverbs played any direct part in the initial argument, but, as gang bosses, both wanted to show their power.

Walker's defending barrister, Philip Valance, QC, didn't attempt to prove his client's innocence: that was out of the question since there were too many witnesses to allow anything but a guilty plea. He told Manchester Crown Court that it had been a 'senseless slaughter' but suggested Walker had not initially intended to kill Proverbs.

His client, he argued, got the gun to 'gain the respect he felt was being denied him . . . but he lost his temper'.

Proverbs was sitting in his HQ, the Spinner's Arms pub, Rolls Crescent, Hulme – subsequently closed – when Walker walked in with three other men. One of the trio and one of Proverbs's cronies had fought over a girl a day or two earlier. Unfortunately the fight had taken place in Walker's flat, which had been damaged in the mêlée, and the young man was said to be 'furious about the invasion of his privacy and the insult to his dignity'.

This might seem rich from a drug dealer not yet past his twenty-second birthday but these men all started their 'adulthood' – making a living and accepting responsibility – much earlier than most. They also knew their lives stood a better chance than most of being spectacularly short.

Proverbs, sitting at the bar, was on his own patch, indeed at the centre of his own world. He probably felt safe but even if he didn't he would never have shown fear. Walker asked him what he was going to do about the furniture broken during the fight involving Proverbs's man. Proverbs replied that he would do nothing.

In these circumstances, in that place, at that time, there was no other answer available to him. To have lost face would have been worse than death. Ridiculously – insanely, to most people's way of thinking – whether he knew it was coming or not, the father of two chose death above dishonour. Walker fired from a range of just a few inches.

When I arrived at the scene Proverbs was lying face up

between a table and a bench, with blood extensively staining the front of his chest. A single gunshot wound had punched a hole one and a quarter inches in diameter in the top of his chest and secondary pellet holes made the total wound area three and a quarter inches.

Proverbs had tattoos on his right forearm, an operation scar on the right lower abdomen from an appendix operation and an old scar on the back of his left hand. Pretty much everything about him was healthy apart from where the shotgun had done its damage.

The larynx was intact but the trachea, just below, was torn across. The lungs were bruised and lacerated at each apex. The pleural cavities contained blood and blood clots and the posterior wall between the first and fourth ribs showed obvious signs of pellet wounds. Several pellets were still in the body. The left common carotid artery had been hit, bleeding into the left side of the neck.

The pellets had entered the lower neck and upper chest in a slightly downward direction, indicating Proverbs had been seated when he died.

The upper part of the sternum and the medial part of the clavical, or breast bone, were destroyed. Damage had occurred to the trachea and oesophagus and the upper part of both lungs, the pellets travelling the full depth of his body.

Proverbs died brutally and instantly for no better reasons than bravado and misplaced pride.

Henderson Proverbs wore his hair in a Rastafarian style, swaggered through his brief life and tried, as those who choose to embrace gang culture often do, to emulate his anti-heroes from TV and the movies. His friends considered him, in today's slang, to be 'seriously cool'. It's cheap irony, I know, but forgive me for recalling that my records show that in the mortuary he was allocated fridge number 20.

Anthony 'Scratch' Gardner was twenty-six, a year older than Henderson Proverbs, when he died. Respect was important to him, too.

He respected his mother and his father, who preached at the United Reformed Church in Chorlton-cum-Hardy, and because he respected them he would never involve them in his life of petty crime or introduce them to someone he knew they would consider improper. Anthony went to church and listened to his father preach.

After he died, like Proverbs, from a single shot to the chest from a sawn-off shotgun, police faced a wall of silence. To this day no one has been charged with the brutal, almost professional killing. Detectives did have a chief suspect but he too was gunned down three years later.

It was January 1988 when Anthony rolled up outside an illegal drinking den or 'shebeen', known in Moss Side as 'Blues'. He was the passenger in a Renault driven by a male dancer friend.

As they braked to a halt in Gretney Walk a man who had been waiting, pacing up and down in the well-lit street but speaking to no one, stepped forward. He pulled a shotgun from under his coat, held it close to his body and fired into the car.

Anthony managed to say: 'I've been shot, get an ambulance.' He crawled over the driver's seat, slid out of the car, tried to stand up and pitched forward onto his face. It took only a minute or two for the preacher's son to die.

At the sound of the shot the club emptied and customers hurled their drugs onto the tarmac of the street, knowing police were on their way. More than £1,000 worth of heroin and cocaine was abandoned like so many sweet wrappers. There were at least fifty people at the establishment but after several days of inquiries the murder-incident team managed to track down just six.

Anthony Gardner was definitely not 'big time' but he ran two girlfriends at any one moment and was liable to go off at the mouth. During this period in Moss Side you didn't need to say much in the wrong place to the wrong people at the wrong time to get swift and terminal retribution.

The post-mortem showed Anthony had lost a massive amount of blood as a consequence of the gunshot wound, indicating that he had not died instantly and that his heart had continued to pump blood out of his body.

The entry wound was two inches in diameter with surrounding pellet patterns increasing the injury area to an uneven circle of about five inches on the left side of the upper chest. The trachea and bronchi contained blood-stained fluid, the pleural cavity on the left side contained blood and blood clot. The wound on the front of the chest had passed through the sterno-clavicular joint and the first left rib. There was a wound in the arch of the aorta, surrounded by an extensive blood clot.

Essentially the shot had taken out the main blood vessels coming from the heart and Anthony had bled to death, not quite instantaneously.

We will probably never know for sure why he was killed – though it is a fair guess that it was not for any worthy reason.

The chief suspect in the murder of Anthony Gardner was a young man who had a remarkable, albeit brief, criminal career.

'White' Tony Johnson – so-called because, while he himself was Caucasian, he led a predominantly Afro-Caribbean gang – would have only been nineteen at the time of that killing. If he was responsible it might have been the event that turned him into the leader of what was known as the Cheetham Hill mob. They were similar to the groups in Moss Side but based on the opposite north side of the city and probably a little better organized. Tony certainly became a fearsome mobster with an almost legendary reputation until his equally brutal and bloody death three years after Anthony's.

Tony was a loose cannon, a Billy the Kid figure who terrified not because of his size or propensity for extreme violence but because of his unpredictability.

Tony sashayed through the city, dealing drugs in nightclubs, notably the famous Hacienda which was temporarily closed down because of his activities. He did what he wanted to do and went where he wanted to go – never paying – simply on his reputation. He felt he was the Prince of the City and was happy to be known as an out-and-out thug. What he wanted he got, no questions asked. Tony, unemployed and the proud owner of a £25,000 Sierra Cosworth, was The Man.

One night at the height of his power in 1991 he agreed to a meeting with people he knew in the car park outside the Penny Black pub, Cheetham Hill. He was with another gangster pal and on his home patch. Rather like doomed Henderson Proverbs, though wary he had no real reason to be particularly worried.

When there are a number of bullet holes in a body the most effective if apparently crude method of matching entry and exit wounds is to run wires through and see where they come out. The results of this on 'White' Tony were straight-forward. They told the story of an individual attempting to escape a clinical attempt at assassination. This was not a killing carried out in anger. This was cold blood.

The men who murdered him knew his capabilities and consequently didn't give him a chance. He saw someone pull a handgun and he started running. I could tell because three of the four bullets that struck him hit him in the back.

The first entered the back of his chest and came out through his mouth and nose. He would have been bent forward in a running crouch when this bullet struck.

The second entered the left side of his back, close to the sixth vertebra, tore through his lung and exited by the second rib. This would have been a fatal wound.

The third hit him in the back of the neck on the left side and came out through the side of his mouth.

Finally, as he lay on the ground, dead or very close to death, the last bullet was fired from close range into his mouth and exited via the top of his right shoulder.

Tony's friend managed to escape the carnage although he too was shot as he ran away. At first he denied any knowledge of who was responsible but some months later named a number of men he claimed had carried out the 'hit'.

Three men, two brothers and a wheelchair-bound cripple who were all associated with the Cheetham gang, knew Tony well and were regarded as his friends, were charged. However, the murdered man's mate was not a particularly convincing witness and one of the three accused had an unshakeable alibi. Two separate juries in two trials failed to reach a majority verdict and the three were formally acquitted.

'White' Tony's killers, whoever they are, have never been

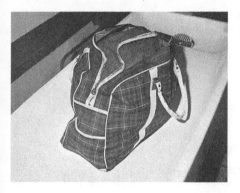

The holdall used to hide Christine Marsh's body.

The hammer used to kill Christine Marsh.

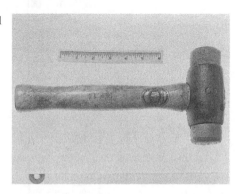

Pauline Reade's white stiletto shoe marking the moors murder victim's shallow grave.

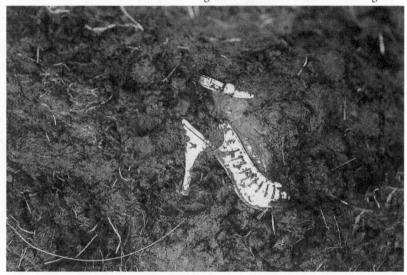

BOEING 737

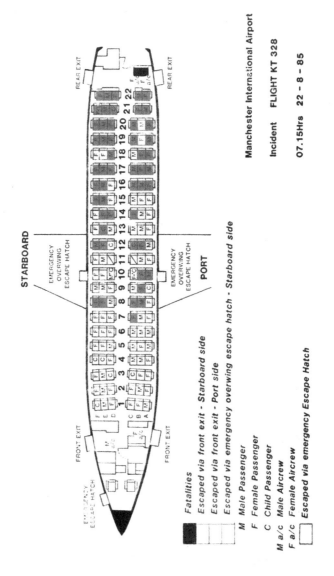

Manchester International Airport

Incident   FLIGHT KT 328

07.15Hrs   22 - 8 - 85

STARBOARD

PORT

EMERGENCY OVERWING ESCAPE HATCH

REAR EXIT
REAR EXIT
FRONT EXIT
FRONT EXIT
EMERGENCY ESCAPE HATCH

Fatalities
Escaped via front exit - Starboard side
Escaped via front exit - Port side
Escaped via emergency overwing escape hatch - Starboard side

M   Male Passenger
F   Female Passenger
C   Child Passenger
M a/c   Male Aircrew
F a/c   Female Aircrew

Escaped via emergency Escape Hatch

The passenger map of the doomed Manchester airport flight to Corfu showing where the fatalities were seated.

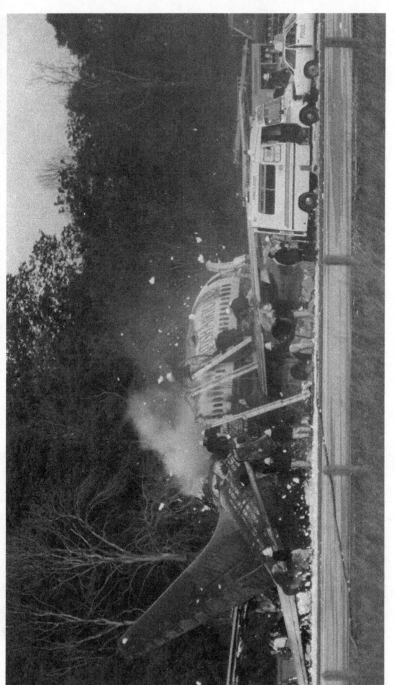

The aftermath of the Manchester Airport disaster.

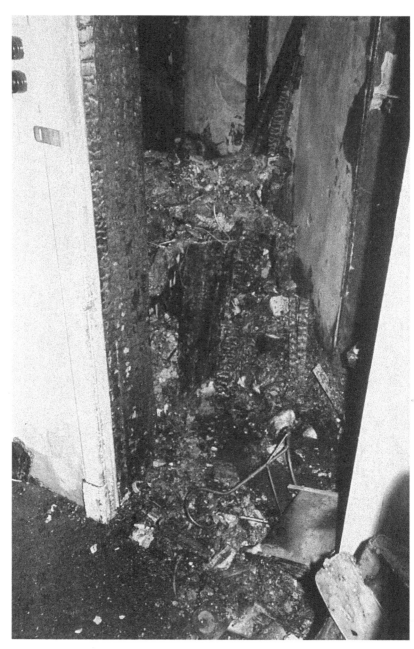

The storeroom at the Mother Mac's pub where the pyre of bodies was found.

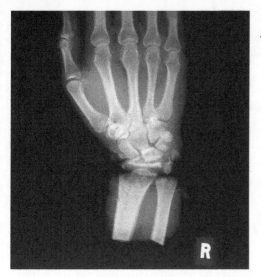

X-ray of drug baron Marty Johnstone's severed hand.

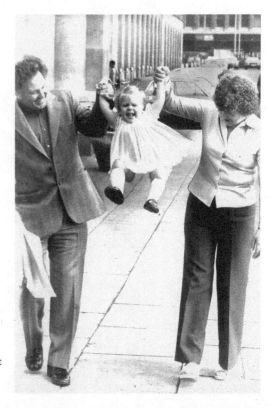

Louise Brown, the world's first 'test-tube baby' born 25 July, 1978.

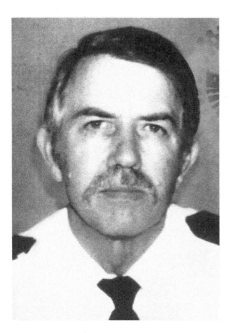

Inspector Ray Codling, shot dead by maniac Anthony Hughes at the M62 Birch service station, Bury, Lancashire.

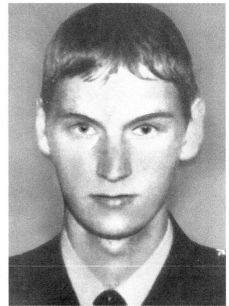

PC John Egerton, stabbed to death in Farnworth, Bolton, by petty crook Arthur Edge on 11 March, 1982.

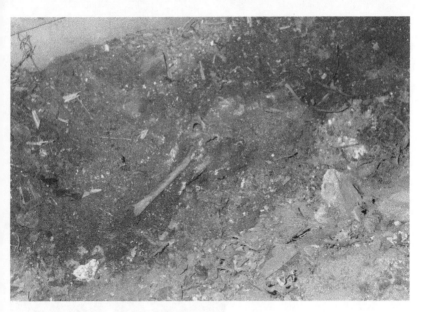

The discovery of skeletal remains in a shallow grave in north Manchester.

The recovered pieces of the skeleton arranged on a table at the mortuary.

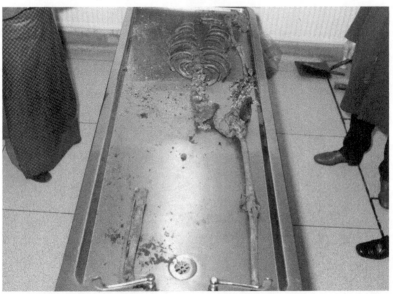

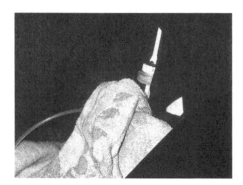

Left and below: DIY abortion kits which killed pregnant women.

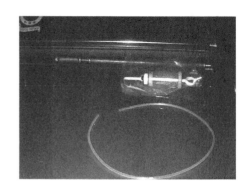

Dr Geoffrey Garrett at work.

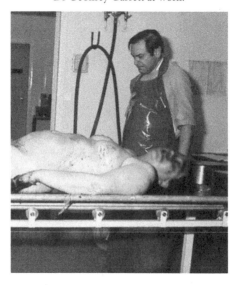

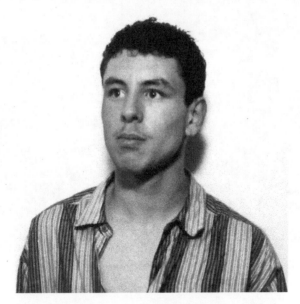

'White' Tony Johnson, gang boss gunned down outside the Penny Black pub in north Manchester.

An X-ray of the shotgun pellets spread through Samuel McDougall's brain.

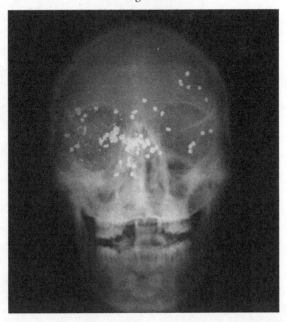

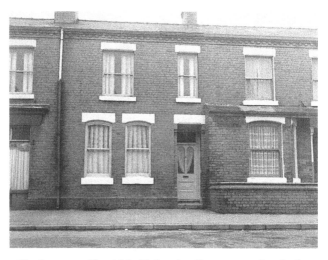

The house outside which Christopher Downey was shot dead.

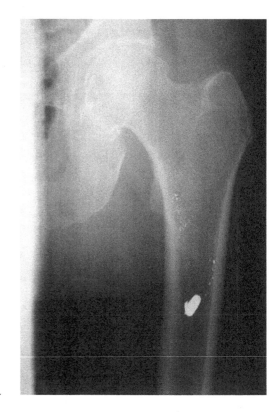

An X-ray of the bullet in Christopher Downey's thigh.

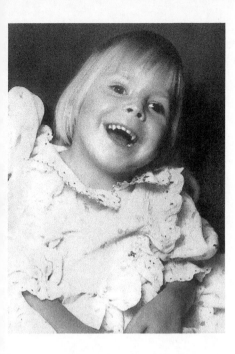

Amanda Jane Allman, aged four. Kevin Callan was convicted of her murder then freed on appeal.

An X-ray of the fatal pellet in Tahir Akram's head.

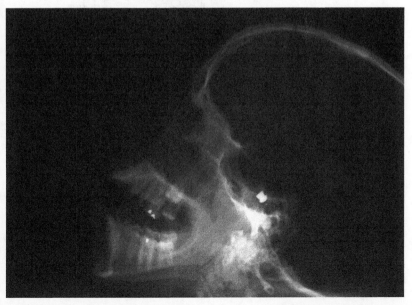

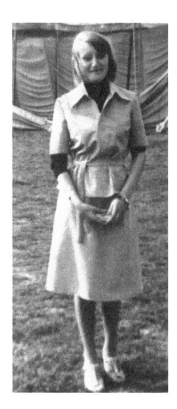

Susan Hockenhull, the bank worker kidnapped and left to freeze to death on a snow-swept moor in Staffordshire.

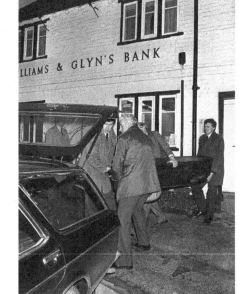

The body of Susan Hockenhull's colleague, Ian Jebb, being removed from Williams and Glyn's Bank in Prestbury, February 1977.

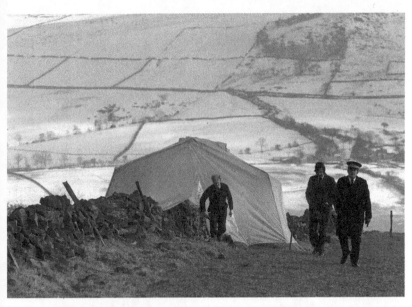

A tent showing the location of Susan Hockenhull's body on the moor.

The Summerland fire on the Isle of Man in which 50 died on 2 August, 1973.

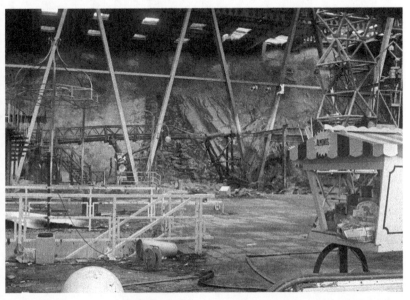

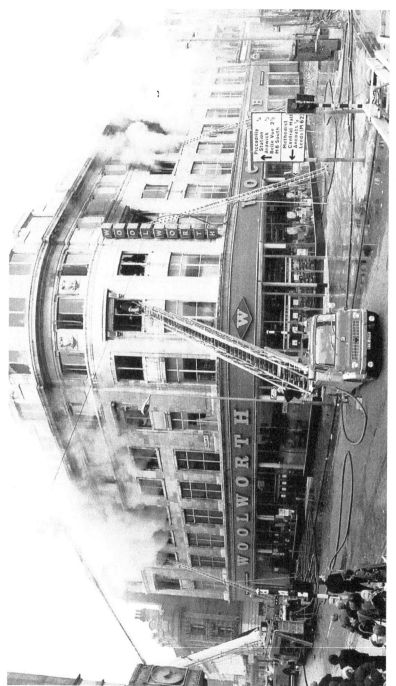

The Woolworths fire, Piccadilly, Manchester, in which 10 died on 8 May, 1979.

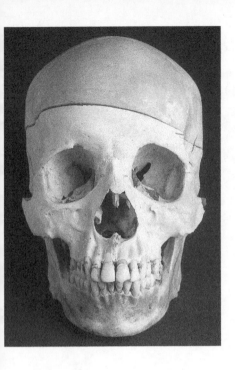

Stages of the re-creation of Sabbir Kilu's face.

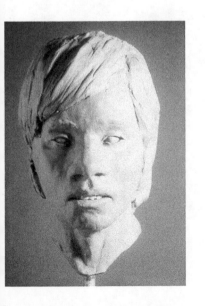

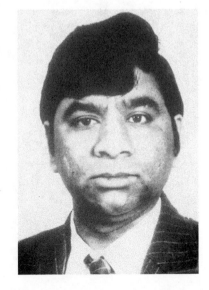

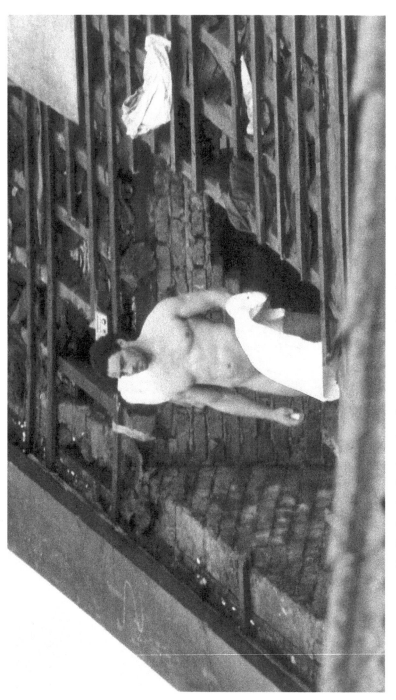

Alan Lord posing for the gathered press cameras on the roof of Strangeways jail, April 1990.

convicted by the system. Perversely, as a man who lived by the sword and fully expected to die by it, it was probably as Tony would have wished.

It is a sad postscript and a strange coincidence that I should twice have become involved with Tony Johnson's family on a professional basis. He was brought up by his grandmother, Winnie, in Fallowfield, Manchester, after being born to her daughter, Susan, when the girl was just fifteen.

Whenever Winnie asked Tony what he was up to he would always say: 'Don't ask, Mum. You don't want to know.'

But before Tony was born, Winnie's twelve-year-old son, Keith Bennett, was killed by the Moors Murderers, Myra Hindley and Ian Brady, and buried on Saddleworth Moor.

Greater Manchester police set up a major operation to try to locate his body and that of Pauline Reade, another victim of the evil pair.

They found Pauline and I carried out the autopsy with a colleague from Yorkshire, details of which are recorded elsewhere in this book, but they never found Keith. Mrs Johnson has had a greater share of tragedy and murder than any mother could reasonably be expected to bear. My heart goes out to her.

Sandra Parhatka was shot to death in September 1988. Although she was neither a gangster nor a drug dealer she was killed because she was part of a society which had grown used to rule by the gun.

A trivial argument was resolved with a shotgun at close range as a team of police officers watched helplessly and in undiluted horror.

Sandra was twenty-six years old, a mother of two and a prostitute. She was a persistent criminal and had been the 'bride' in at least five bogus marriages designed to help mostly African men beat the British immigration laws.

One evening while Sandra was working on Chorlton Road, Old Trafford, wearing a distinctive red miniskirt and black leather jacket, she was approached by a man she knew. We can assume that at that moment she wasn't afraid.

As three police officers watched from an unmarked car 140 yards away, the conversation became strained and Sandra turned away from the man. The police knew she was a prostitute and would have assumed that there had been some haggling over price. They did not expect anything dramatic to happen.

But as they looked on in sickened disbelief they saw the man pull something from under his coat. Then there was blast of flame and a bang. The girl fell down like a rag doll.

In the seconds that it took the police to get to her the man had made his escape. They found Sandra desperately injured and, as it turned out, twenty-five minutes from inevitable death.

The wound caused by the pellets was horizontal. It entered the left side of the neck, causing a one-and-a-half-inch-diameter wound just above the clavical and destroyed the cervical spine. That Sandra did not die instantly was perhaps surprising. She certainly had no chance of survival whatever the police officers or the doctors in Casualty did.

Days later unemployed Kenneth Alexander, thirty-eight, was arrested and charged with killing Sandra. At first he denied any involvement but eventually he pleaded guilty to manslaughter. He claimed he believed that

Sandra had been involved in the theft of his girlfriend's video recorder and had only intended to frighten her. His explanation was that his tie had somehow caught on the trigger mechanism and had caused the weapon to discharge accidentally.

The evidence of the police witnesses and my opinion that the girl was moving away from him at the time, based on the direction of the shot through the body, helped the jury to find him guilty of murder.

Quite simply, there is never any reason for anyone to carry a loaded shotgun unless, of course, they intend to use it to kill someone or something. Sandra died as much from the culture of the gun that existed in inner-city Manchester at the time as she did from the action of a stupid, violent man.

The gun-lobby suggestion that 'guns don't kill people, people kill people' is obnoxious self-serving garbage. Most of the time an angry man is just a nuisance. But give him a weapon, particularly a gun, and he becomes a menace.

If Alexander had gone out that night to frighten Sandra Parhatka without a weapon she might have got beaten up and he still might have gone to jail. But she would almost certainly not have died.

People kill people, that is true. But guns make it a damned sight easier.

While judges and barristers are, of course, integral to our system of justice, they are all, much to their chagrin, junior to the jury, particularly if the twelve good persons and true are feeling lenient.

Should someone be found guilty they can appeal against their conviction and sentence and a sensible senior judge can either release them or cut their jail term.

He can also increase the prison sentence, but in practice this happens only rarely. Any lawyer who takes you to Appeal only for you to see your sentence increased needs to go back to law school.

But should a jury acquit, that's it. No matter what anyone feels or believes, the individual is not guilty.

Sometimes the accused can be acquitted of the most heinous charge for reasons other than the facts of the case. It could be their demeanour, the demeanour of some of his accusers in the witness box, or it could be that the jury chooses to take a wider view.

The well-publicized case of the women who broke into a British Aerospace plant in Preston and wrecked a fighter plane is a case in point. Clearly they were guilty of criminal damage but the jury was swayed by an ideological defence argument that the women's actions prevented slaughter in the Far East, as that was where the aircraft was destined. In law it was a fragile defence but in front of the right jury it proved to be brilliant and successful. They were acquitted. And that was that.

Further, a jury does not need to give reasons or provide excuses for its judgements: the group simply reaches its verdict, which is absolutely binding in law. If that verdict goes against the evidence, the common good, or even the judge's summing up, then so be it.

Grocer Mansukhlal Pankhania is not a murderer. He killed a man by shooting him at point-blank range with a shotgun but he is not a murderer. A jury at Manchester Crown Court decided he was guilty of manslaughter. The judge, clearly in agreement, gave him a two-year suspended sentence. The guilty man walked free from court with the judge's praises ringing in his ears.

I believe he was very fortunate to do so and perhaps benefited from the mood of society prevailing at the time. The killer was a shopkeeper in Moss Side, the victim a burglar clearly intent on his chosen trade who was in the shop out of hours when he died.

Many people hold the view that burglars deserve all they get and perhaps shooting a few of them isn't such a bad way forward. I wonder if any of them were on this jury.

Mr Pankhania, twenty-six, from Little Lever, Bolton, had suffered abominably at the hands of thieves. His shop in Timwood Walk was constantly targeted by burglars and it seemed to him that the police could do little to protect his business.

This was in 1979, two years before the Moss Side riots and a period when many people, especially ethnic-minority communities, felt abandoned by the authorities.

Mr Pankhania got hold of a shotgun and lay in wait for the next burglar.

In evidence the gunman said he got the weapon to 'scare intruders'. His next intruder was a twenty-year-old local thief with a string of convictions called Samuel McDougall. An ambulance took him to hospital but he was dead on arrival.

At the mortuary I found a single entry wound at the left ear. It was a fairly tight hole, less than two inches in diameter, suggesting a range of certainly less than three yards, the length of a decent-sized sofa.

The shot had entered his cranium and effectively obliterated his brain. There was no exit wound. All the pellets simply ricocheted around in his head until they stopped. Samuel would have known nothing at all about it.

The position of entry, at the back of the ear, told me that

McDougall had already turned away from his assailant before the gun was fired. Assuming the two men had confronted each other face to face, McDougall had completed 120 degrees of a 180-degree turn when he was fired upon.

My immediate thought, without the benefit of any testimony from the parties involved, was that he had been killed while in the process of retreating, which certainly rules out any suggestion of self-defence and usually results in a verdict of murder.

Mr Pankhania insisted it had been an accident. He explained in court that when the burglar, who was carrying a screwdriver, broke in, he, Pankhania, was 'shaking and frightened'. McDougall, he said, raised his hand as if to throw something but the gun went off. Pankhania steadfastly insisted he did not intend the weapon to fire.

After the manslaughter verdict the judge, Mr Justice Caulfield, described Pankhania as a man of 'impeccable character, hard-working and law-abiding'.

He added: 'I am sure everyone in this court has the greatest sympathy for you regarding the battering your business endured, particularly in the week before the killing.'

While I do have every sympathy for anyone who suffers the trauma of a burglary, I do wonder about what exactly happened in that jury room and what the arguments were.

In 1979 burglary was not a capital offence.

Like Sandra Parhatka, like Tony Johnson, Henderson Proverbs, Anthony Gardner and so many others, Samuel McDougall died because someone who was angry had access to a gun.

He would not have been killed, accidentally or otherwise,

but for that one fact. The argument for banning guns is simple and unequivocal. They have no place in civilized society.

On the other hand, for several years they kept me in work.

10

The Irish Connection

Many people have lived to regret going to the newspapers with their stories. Christopher Downey lived twenty-nine days.

The Irishman contacted the *News of the World* and offered to tell how he had been kidnapped and tortured by the IRA. Within a month a masked gunman appeared at his door and fired eight shots from a Browning .22 target pistol.

Downey was forty-one years old, a ladies' man, a suspected terrorist – and my first gunshot-murder victim.

I was, to say the least, apprehensive about dealing with a shooting. In the autumn of 1973 guns were still a rarity on British streets. I didn't really know what to expect or how to act, although, on arrival at the murder scene, I felt I should be doing something to instil confidence in those around me.

The police were in a similar situation since few of them had ever been involved in the investigation of a gun murder.

Fortunately, help was close at hand in the shape of Jim Biggs, a bluff, likeable and, most importantly, highly experienced forensic scientist who had also been called out on the job.

It was clear to me that he had taken charge of the situation because the senior officers were staying well back while he went through his obviously well-practised routine.

It was 1.30 a.m. and Ackroyd Street, Openshaw, Manchester, had been sealed off. The police had got lights to illuminate the body, which was lying face down. I could see that the shirt and vest were bloodstained and there was more blood on the ground beneath the dead man.

Jim was prowling around the grim scene like a tiger, moving from one vantage point to another. Starting from the head, he moved in an anticlockwise direction around to the side and then to the feet and around once more to the head, completing 360 degrees, taking it all in. He'd stop, notice something, appraise the situation, give it time to make sense in his own very logical fashion, log it in his mind for notation, then start again, his face a picture of concentration, brow furrowed, eyes narrowed. Focused. Everyone left the expert alone to do his work. Interruption was unthinkable.

When the spell was finally broken and he looked up and saw me he smiled an acknowledgement. I stepped the few paces forward to join him, awaiting instructions.

After a brief silence, I assumed in respect for the dead man, he took a breath while still looking down at the corpse and whispered conspiratorially out of the side of his mouth so no one else could hear, 'What do we do now, Geoff? This is my first shooting.'

Christopher Downey had abandoned his home in the New Lodge area of Belfast after falling foul of both sides of the Ulster conflict. He was arrested by the Army after suspicions arose that he was a member of C Company of the Provisional IRA's Third Belfast Brigade. After twenty-four hours' questioning at Girwood barracks he was released without charge.

Later Downey was picked up by IRA men and beaten in

a punishment ritual. He argued afterwards that when the Provos released him they told him they had made a mistake and got the wrong man.

He told his girlfriend, Annie Gibson, that he had been picked up by two men in a car and taken to a secret hideout where he had been kept in a wardrobe for two days and only let out for beatings. Finally a tin of paint was thrown over him.

This was a mild form of the tar-and-feather punishment, which suggested that he was suspected of committing a misdemeanour in the eyes of the IRA rather than a genuinely serious wrong. Nevertheless, it scared him out of the Province and into Manchester where Annie had family.

The couple returned to Ulster just twice: once in March 1972 to visit Annie's son, Edward, in hospital after he had been shot in the leg for allegedly being an Army informer, and then in July that same year for the funeral of Downey's nephew Joseph, twenty-five, who had been shot dead by the Army as a suspected terrorist. While the question of which side he truly supported was never clear, the idea that Downey was terrorist-connected made a lot of sense.

He drank a lot and when he drank he talked a lot. Often that talk was of the IRA and how much he knew about the organization. Sometimes he spoke of getting revenge for the beating he didn't deserve. Often he threatened to go to the newspapers. On 21 September he was as good as his word and telephoned the *News of the World* office in Manchester.

Asking for no money, Downey offered to name names and expose the terrorists for 'the bullies they are'. He made no secret of the fact that he had spoken to a journalist but three days later rang the paper back to cancel the planned detailed interview. He said he had had second thoughts.

On Sunday, 22 October he and Annie went out for the evening, first to the Oldfield pub and then to the Bridge Inn on Abbey Hey Lane, Gorton. They were there until closing time at 10.30 p.m. and stayed chatting with friends outside until 11 p.m.

It was a short walk home to Ackroyd Street. As they approached the house Downey was just a little ahead and to the left of his girlfriend. He had the door key in his hand when he heard footsteps from behind and turned to see a man running out of the shadows towards the two of them.

As the gun's muzzle flashed Downey pushed Annie to one side and the bullet hit the door. Downey shouted: 'You bastard,' and the shooter stopped in his tracks and began to turn. Perhaps encouraged by the other man's apparent change of heart, perhaps impelled by sheer rage, Downey made the fatal mistake of giving chase.

Moments later, cut down in a hail of bullets, he managed to stagger back into Annie's arms and died as she held him.

There were four distinct bullet holes on the trunk of the body, another two in the left arm and one in the left buttock.

Bullets were found in the muscles at the back of the chest and in the abdominal cavity. The heart had escaped direct damage but there was clotted blood in the pericardial sac that encloses the heart and which had been pierced by the track of one bullet passing through the upper end of the pericardium.

There were two bullet holes in the upper lobes of both lungs and one in the lower lobe of the left lung. There were further holes in each cusp of the diaphragm and extensive bleeding in the left pleural cavity.

Downey died of internal haemorrhage caused by gunshots.

An examination of the bullets and cartridge cases found at the scene and in the body showed they were .22-calibre Eley rifle bullets, common target ammunition, and had probably been fired from a Browning ten-shot self-loading pistol. Three entrance holes in the left front of the victim's topcoat showed the presence of powder residues, indicating a range of between twelve and twenty-four inches. Downey had got very close to his killer.

Details of the bullets were forwarded to the Data Reference Centre in Belfast and the Metropolitan Police forensic laboratory.

Police were disappointed with the response from the public when they launched their murder inquiry. While there was no proof of terrorist involvement word quickly spread that it was the work of the Provos – their first assassination on the mainland – and many people were simply too scared to come forward.

No one was ever charged with the murder. But four years later the gun that was used in the killing was recovered from a house forty miles away in Moreton on the Wirral.

Routine ballistic checks matched the records sent to Belfast and London. However, no evidence ever came to light that might have linked the holder of the weapon, a taxi driver who said it had been left in his cab, with Downey's murder.

Nowadays, with the Irish peace process understandably considered more important than any police investigation into IRA affairs, one might be cynical about the inquiry's findings. However, at that time in the 1970s it is unlikely that there was any political reason to protect the killer of Christopher Downey or, indeed, to consider the matter of his death in anything other than a straightforward investigative manner.

The man who committed this murder escaped justice. Looking at his apparently amateur *modus operandi*, it was most likely his first killing. We don't know if it was his last.

11

An Appealing Man

In January 1992 Kevin John Callan was convicted of murdering his girlfriend's doll-sized handicapped daughter, a girl of four called Amanda Jane Allman. She had twenty-five separate injuries, most of them recent. Her death was caused by a cerebral haemorrhage that, in my opinion, was of a type consistent with her having been violently shaken. I found bruises on both sides of her brain indicating that her head had moved rapidly in more than one direction, the momentum bringing her brain into hard contact with her skull.

In prison, the lorry driver who had left school without a single GCSE spent much of his time reading books on the subject of brain damage. He occupied long hours and days writing letters to doctors around the world, notably to a neurologist in New Zealand, Dr Phillip Wrightson, who had written a book called *Head Injuries – the Facts*, which Callan had acquired in prison.

Within a relatively brief time this uneducated man became startlingly well versed in what is, by any standards, a complex field of medicine. This, however, was not a morbid fixation, not the behaviour of a killer obsessively trying to understand the medical aspects of the act of violence that caused him to be punished. Kevin Callan was working on his defence.

His argument in court was that he never attacked the dead girl and he assumed she must have received the injuries from falling from a slide in the garden. Although the jury felt otherwise and unanimously found him guilty he steadfastly stuck to his position and consistently insisted he was an innocent man.

In 1995, just four years after Amanda Jane's death, and three after Callan's conviction, Dr Wrightson, the Antipodean author, stated that, in his expert opinion, the child's injuries could have been caused in the accidental manner the prisoner contended. As a direct consequence of this 'new evidence' the Court of Appeal found that the verdict was 'unsafe' and released Callan.

The case attracted a great deal of publicity and the newly freed 'medical student' briefly enjoyed celebrity status for achieving his freedom through undertaking this remarkable act of study from inside jail. It was newsworthy enough that Callan was capable of becoming an expert neurologist when forced to carry out his research with the limited facilities of life in a cell. But that his newfound knowledge led to release from an unjust sentence for a child murder was truly sensational.

This was the stuff of movies. Where was David Puttnam?

Of course, such a result did not reflect well on me. Enough significant doubt had been cast upon my findings for a man convicted of a capital crime to be set free. My position as an expert witness and my professional competence were put in question. Suddenly, *I* was the person in the dock.

Whether Callan was innocent or guilty is not for me to say. The jury had found him guilty but the Appeal judges felt there were grounds for that verdict to be considered unsafe. Whether justice was served or not, Callan's defence ultimately prevailed over the prosecution's. That is what a defence is for: it is the due process of law. Callan is now a free man and will remain so for ever in respect of this matter.

However, now is the time for me to set out my own defence.

What I say from this point on is not intended in any way to be a retrial of a man accused and then found innocent of murder. The legal case is concluded and cannot be reopened. But I do certainly feel I have been let down by the forensic establishment, some of whom have subsequently chosen to express fresh doubts about shaking being one cause of brain damage. They should look at the damage inflicted upon boxers' brains, a subject dealt with elsewhere in this book, before they lightly dismiss this means of harm.

All that to one side, this is a review of evidence with which I was associated. It is also my attempt to show that my conclusion that the young girl's death was non-accidental was, within the bounds of reasonable doubt, the most likely scenario. I believe it is only fair in the circumstances that I should take this opportunity to present my own 'new evidence', information available at the time of the trial that backed up my point of view but which the jury was not allowed to hear for numerous reasons of law that are there to ensure a fair trial for the accused.

The jury, as it turned out, did not require this evidence to find Callan guilty and it was not offered for study to the Court of Appeal, so from that point of view it is irrelevant. However, it does strengthen my own personal and professional defence and since Callan is now, and will remain, a free man, it can no longer prejudice his case.

At the Appeal hearing the eminent barrister representing Callan, Mr Richard Henriques, QC, took steps to damn my own professional reputation while enhancing the perceived character of his client. Importantly for his case, for his client and, as it turned out, for me, he insisted to the judges that my opinion had been contradicted by every other doctor consulted. That was possibly the most important and compelling statement made during the hearing. It effectively isolated me within the forensic-pathology community. It was a statement that marked me as a pariah. It was also untrue.

Here is the proof.

It was on the afternoon of Tuesday, 16 April 1991 that I was called to the mortuary at Tameside Hospital, Ashton-Under-Lyne, and shown the body of a four-year-old girl.

Amanda Jane Allman had been dead on her arrival in Casualty. When Dr Freeman, the consultant paediatrician, examined her, he found that her body bore a large number of injuries of different ages that were, in his opinion, consistent with the little girl having been seriously physically abused on several different occasions over a period of about a week. He believed the assaults, for that was what he was convinced these marks were evidence of, had involved severe shaking and punching.

He was also of the opinion that the injuries were totally inconsistent with the explanation that had been offered, which was that she had fallen from a children's slide onto a grassy surface.

The hospital had called in the police and the police had called in me. I carried out a post-mortem examination with Dr Freeman present.

I found that Amanda Jane was small for her age and

underdeveloped. I was told that she suffered from cerebral palsy that had been diagnosed at about the age of nine months.

There were bruises on her forehead and left cheek, close to the left eye. At least seven bruises were visible over the front of the left side of her chest and upper abdomen. There was further bruising in the right groin and multiple bruises present on the front of both her legs. On the back of her head was a small laceration and she had ill-defined bruises on her back. I counted twenty-five separate injuries.

Internally, the significant findings were blood clots over both cerebral hemispheres and a swelling of the brain. There was some bruising of the front of the scalp but no fracture of the skull. There were some abdominal injuries but these were consistent with the attempts at resuscitation that would have been made either by an ambulance crew or by hospital staff on arrival at casualty.

Dr Freeman told me that he had examined the child's eyes and found that both contained retinal haemorrhages suggesting a bleed from the brain. The post-mortem findings confirmed his clinical diagnosis of intracranial bleeding probably due to a subdural haematoma. He believed the likeliest cause was a direct blow or a vigorous shake. I have examined children on a number of occasions after they have died because they were violently shaken. This fitted that pattern in all respects. I agreed with Dr Freeman's opinion and concluded that the cause of death was a cerebral haemorrhage consistent with violent shaking.

A week later I visited the mortuary once again, this time to watch another doctor perform a post-mortem on Amanda Jane. In criminal cases it is normal practice for a second post-mortem to be carried out on behalf of the defence and customary that the first pathologist be invited to observe.

Dr S. Variend, a consultant from the Children's Hospital in Sheffield, was shown the photographs taken at the original examination and was able to confirm what they showed on the body. He further discovered a chain of recent ill-defined bruises running on either side of the lumbar spine. These could have been produced by the fingers of an individual holding the little girl tightly with his hands around her abdomen or chest. She was small enough for someone to reach nearly all the way around with two hands.

Dr Variend's conclusions matched mine. His report stated: 'The brain swelling and haemorrhage resulted probably from violent shaking of the head on the shoulders. For this type of injury to be produced it would have required an adult to hold the body of the child around the chest or abdomen in a tight grip while at the same time producing vigorous to-and-fro movements. This would have caused the head to rock backwards and forwards on the shoulders, resulting in marked disruptive forces within and around the brain.

'Alternatively, a direct blow or blows to the head with the flat of the hand or a fisted hand or even a kick might be expected to produce a similar injury. Of course, a fall from a height on to a hard, unyielding surface associated with a type of whiplash injury to the head is another explanation.' This was a consideration of the possibility that the head had hit the ground and, as a consequence, the brain had bounced within the skull on impact, creating a bruise on the other side, i.e. two bruises from the same fall.

However, the paediatrician went on: 'In considering the possibility of either of the last two mechanisms, it is important to remember that the bruises around the head were generally at least a day or more old and therefore unlikely to have been concerned directly with the cause of death. The one exception was the bruise at the outer aspect of the left eye which appeared to be reasonably fresh.

'It is, of course, quite possible that the bruising around the head was temporally disassociated [happened at a different time] and consequently additional to the shaking injury. A shaking injury would have required gripping around the torso; that this had actually occurred here is supported by what are possibly rows of fingertip bruising involving the skin over the back on either side of the spine.'

The specialist also stated that he would find it very difficult to explain Amanda Jane's brain injury by a fall from a children's slide.

He was not called to give evidence at the trial by the defence. Although the police were aware of his conclusions the prosecution was not able to insist that he should appear because he was a defence witness. That is the law.

The defence turned to a consultant paediatrician from Liverpool, Dr John Sills, who had experience in childhood diseases and had worked for two and a half years in paediatric neurology, dealing with many forms of neurological handicap in children, including cerebral palsy.

In his conclusions he referred to one of the post-mortem photographs and stated: 'The photograph shows the collection of subdural blood [blood collecting under the outer membrane of the brain] which would be most likely to be due to a shaking injury rather than a direct blow in the absence of a skull fracture. Retinal haemorrhages as described by Dr Freeman are probably due to the same shaking force.'

Dr Sills also dismissed a fall from a slide as a likely cause of the girl's injuries, adding: 'It appears clear that Amanda was another victim of child abuse, i.e. that her death was due to non-accidental injuries. Dr Garrett did not find a skull fracture and his conclusion that the subdural haemorrhage was due to severe shaking would be appropriate in the circumstances.'

Despite the cost of paying Dr Sills to study the case and reach conclusions, once again the defence chose not to call him to give his expert-witness evidence at the trial.

I took the stand on Wednesday, 15 January 1992 and was rigorously questioned by Jack Price, QC, the defence counsel. I felt he did a good job but, looking back, I consider that I was firm in my stance and he was unable to shake me in my contention that these were non-accidental injuries. Professor Michael Green, the pathologist from Yorkshire with whom I worked on the Pauline Reade Moors case, was later to say that he thought from his reading of the transcripts of the court case that I had been given 'an easy time' by the defence. He was not there and I maintain he is wrong. There are suggestions that I had been too dogmatic. Again, I disagree. At the most I was firm. In any case, I was clearly acceptable to the jury.

It has been said since that my evidence was the main reason for Callan's conviction and, of course, a later discrediting of my evidence and my evidence alone was sufficient for him to be set free.

But the jury heard from other witnesses as well and it should be remembered that all I stated was that I believed the child had died as the result of an attack. That was all. It was never part of my evidence that Callan was the individual responsible. The members of the jury made that decision without me and it is interesting to note some of the things they were asked to consider during their deliberations.

They were advised that Amanda Jane was born on 14 April 1987, at Ashton-under-Lyne to Lesley Sharon Bridgewood and Darrell Allman. They had a second daughter, Natalie, eighteen months later. But the relationship fell apart and they split up in March 1990, with the children remaining with their mother.

Amanda's cerebral palsy had been diagnosed when she was nine months old and her condition left her small for her age and only capable of walking between six and nine steps at a time. In January 1990 she started at the Child Development Unit at Poplar Street Primary School.

Teachers said she was outgoing, bubbly, extrovert and happy with adults. She was unable to speak words but was capable of laughter and her initial progress at the nursery was described as satisfactory. Hope was expressed for her future as she was keen to work and cooperative with the staff. It was an optimistic picture.

In September that year, six months after the split with Amanda Jane's father, Kevin Callan moved into the house in Peel Street, Hyde, that the four-year-old shared with her mother.

During three weeks of that month the little girl was looked after by family friends while Lesley was in Portugal. Throughout this period the teachers said the child became upset and this was put down to her mother being away. However, some felt it went deeper than that.

They noticed a marked change in her personality: she was not so outgoing and started crying towards the end of the day at school, apparently not wanting to go home. On occasions, the jury was told, Amanda Jane became hysterical, clinging on to members of staff. During the early months of 1991 her attendance at school was good. Small bruises were noticed but these were consistent with simple falls.

However, on Monday, 8 April it was noted that she had severe bruising to her left jaw and inside her left arm and she could not bear weight on her left leg. Concerned, Tameside Borough Council social services made arrangements for Amanda to be medically examined.

Dr Lorraine Lorrence conducted the examination and found that an injury to the child's face and a bruise to her left thigh could have occurred from a fall. However, she was not satisfied about the causes of other bruises and called for a case conference with social workers.

On Thursday, 11 April a cab called to take Amanda to school. Callan met the driver at the door and informed him that she would not be going that day. She failed to make it the day after as well.

The driver, in his evidence, explained that he had conveyed Amanda to and from the special unit attached to the school every day since January of 1991. Over the period he got to know and like the friendly, cheerful youngster and said she was, despite her obvious disabilities, bright and happy. However, from the time he began to notice a man at her home her mood, he said, changed. And, he told the jury, when the man came to lift her out of the taxi on her return from school, she would start crying.

Seven hours before Amanda was declared dead, a social worker called to make a regular check on the child. She was informed by Callan, who said he was alone in the house, that the child was well and sleeping upstairs. When the little girl's mother returned home from a hospital visit she found him screaming and attempting resuscitation on the child's limp body.

This is background, circumstantial evidence not in any way intended by me to point a finger at anyone. However, I believe it is fair to suggest that this is the sort of information that might influence a jury, irrespective of any medical evidence. In other words, though it is fair to state that my pathological evidence was indeed very pertinent to the case, it was never the *whole* of the case. To say that my opinion *alone* convicted Kevin Callan is mistaken. We pathologists don't have that kind of power.

Shortly after I retired early in 1992 I was contacted by Home Office pathologist Dr Helen Whitwell who had been asked to take another look at the case by Callan's lawyers. I suggested that she should speak to Dr Variend as he had the requisite slides.

Two years later I received a copy of a report that she had prepared for the defence in which she made a number of adverse comments about my own original pathological examination report.

Dr Whitwell complained about my description of the body. However, everything I described was supported by photographs, which are far more valuable and accurate than a verbose description.

She referred to the fact that the brain was not placed in formalin prior to dissection to 'fix' it, i.e. dry it out to make it easier to view. However, that is a process which takes weeks and is not really necessary if no cerebral lesions [injuries] are apparent during the external examination of the brain. So-called 'wet cutting', which can be carried out immediately, allows for better examination of surface

209

haemorrhages as it easier to wash away the fresh blood and, should lesions be found, the process can be stopped and the slices fixed for later examination. Furthermore, if I had detected any traumatic lesion on the surface of the brain it would have helped Callan in his insistence that there had been a fall.

So my problem at the time was to decide whether I should examine the brain straightaway and provide the police with their information, bearing in mind that another doctor had already suggested the girl had been criminally injured, or whether I should instead insist that they should wait for several weeks to get the same result. I went ahead and found no external lesion, consequently concluding that shaking had been a more likely cause of Amanda's injuries than a direct blow.

Dr Whitwell continued stating that she felt that at four years of age Amanda was outside the normal age range in the majority of child-shaking cases. This is true, but she failed to take into account the unusual nature of development caused by the girl's cerebral palsy. As Professor Michael Green, from Sheffield, another eminent consultant asked to consider the case, pointed out: 'I accept that Amanda is outside the usual age group in which fatal non-accidental injuries occur. However, her weight was that of a girl of eighteen months and her height that of a girl of about two years. If one accepts the old paediatric law – that young children are abused because they are small enough to abuse – then Amanda fits quite nicely within the parameters.'

I also received a report by Dr Wrightson, the New Zealand-based neurosurgeon, that outlined the clinical history, summarized the prosecution case and then criticized it. His alternative scenario offered the proposition that two injuries occurring within a short time of each other could have a cumulative effect similar to that which I found. Callan had told him the child had fallen twice, once from a swing and on another occasion down the stairs.

I still believe this was the defence clutching at straws. Professor Green, who had been asked by the Crown Prosecution Service to get involved, was presented with the same papers the defence's experts had worked from and asked to prepare a report. He was also made aware that other witnesses in the trial had provided a background that suggested the possibility of child abuse. He said: 'Medical evidence is nearly always a matter of possibilities and probabilities rather than absolute proof beyond reasonable doubt, and this applies in this case.'

Those are sentiments with which I totally agree but, crucially, Professor Green went on to recommend to the CPS in his report: 'I feel that this Appeal [by Callan against his conviction] should be opposed.'

Later Professor Green consulted colleagues in paediatric neurology and paediatric ophthalmology who both took the view that the presence of retinal haemorrhages is diagnostic of a severe head injury but is not seen in children who have suffered a fall through a short distance or even in child road-accident victims.

On Thursday, 6 April 1995 Kevin John Callan walked out of jail and into the arms of a fascinated Press that, understandably enough in the circumstances, treated him like a hero and unilaterally accepted his innocence.

They accepted that he must have been right, that Amanda Jane had died after injuring herself in two falls, one from a slide and one down the stairs. Both falls were accidents and not acts of violence. I repeat Professor Green's words: 'Medical evidence is nearly always a matter of possibilities and probabilities rather than absolute proof beyond reasonable doubt.' My opinion then is my opinion now: this little girl died from non-accidental injury. However, I could be mistaken, of course. I do not claim infallibility. I would not now, and did not ever say that shaking was the only and absolute cause of death. I said it was singularly the most likely, based upon my experience of similar events. If I was wrong then I am deeply sorry for I helped put an innocent man in prison. But I can only give conclusions as I honestly find them.

Stretching the possibilities even further, there may even be a so-far-undiscovered reason involving another unidentified individual that led to the death of this child, someone who arrived either unseen or with connivance, committed murder and left. It has happened before.

However, it is unlikely. The record shows that my findings, matched with the testimony of those who had had contact with Amanda Jane, led police to believe that Kevin John Callan was responsible and, accordingly, he was charged with her murder.

After a long process of law he was released and, in front of the clicking shutters of dozens of Press cameras, ran straight into the arms of his girlfriend, Lesley, Amanda Jane's mother, who had stuck by him throughout.

As far as I know they are still together.

It would surely be difficult for a man who had killed a child to return to that youngster's mother as a loving companion. It would take a person of remarkable callousness to act the innocent every hour of every day while looking into the eyes of a mother robbed by him of a lovely, though oh-so-vulnerable daughter. How could any remotely normal human being live with such a terrible burden?

By the same token, mothers have remarkable instincts when it comes to their offspring. The bond is so close as to sometimes appear almost supernatural. You would think that in such a situation one would be able to tell. Surely she would just know!

Perhaps that also adds to the case for the defence.

For his sake I hope Kevin John Callan's conscience is clear.

Mine is.

12

Man's Inhumanity
to Woman

Like Trevor Joseph Hardy, Peter Sullivan was a loser, a jailbird and a man with few friends. However, until one horrific summer night in 1986, no one suspected him capable of extreme violence.

As a boy he was troublesome and was bullied. He was easily scared and so, naturally, boys picked on him. Boys are like that. Once he was forced to swallow metal nuts and bolts.

He was never bright and probably a little backward. His chances of achieving anything worthwhile were about nil but he dreamed of being a success. Living in a typically 'Walter Mitty' world, he boasted of being friendly with his heroes, world darts champions Eric Bristow and Jocky Wilson. Another time he claimed to have had soccer trials with Wolverhampton Wanderers. While in Risley prison, Warrington, awaiting trial for murder, he insisted he was passing the time by studying for GCSE Maths and English. None of it was true.

The boy stole from his own parents in Oxton, Wirral, Cheshire, swiping electrical goods and selling them down the road. His parents told the police but it didn't stop him. They never kept radios long.

Before the killing Sullivan had accumulated eighteen convictions for minor offences, mostly petty thefts and stealing cars, and had been sentenced to a total of five years in prison.

Once he smashed a window and just stood there, waiting to be caught. Another time his stolen car broke down so he stopped a policeman to help him get it started again. The policeman arrested him. The only way Sullivan could get attention was by misbehaving and being caught misbehaving. Here, surely, was one of life's victims.

Somehow he persuaded an older woman to live with him and they had a child. But he only worked on and off for six years before being finally sentenced at the age of thirty to life imprisonment.

The one thing Sullivan wasn't bad at was darts. He was far from good, certainly not as talented as his father and younger brother – that was the story of his life – but he had a fair eye and a steady arm and was good enough on his day for a pub team.

The night of the murder was also the night Sullivan played his first official match for the darts team of the Crown Hotel on Conway Street, Birkenhead. He lost. He drank heavily from 7.30 p.m. and, after his disappointing match, he joined a group of regulars in another game of darts. Prophetically, they played 'killer'.

At 11.30 p.m. he downed the last of his pint and staggered out of the pub, down Conway Street and back to his maisonette in nearby Queensbury Gardens. There, for reasons we don't know, he picked up a two-foot-long iron crowbar he had borrowed from a friend, stuffed it uncomfortably inside his jacket, went back out again and wandered half a mile to Borough Road, Birkenhead.

A few minutes earlier a twenty-one-year-old woman ran out of petrol and rolled her Fiat van to a stop on a roundabout in the town. Diane Sindall, a pretty, likeable lass, was scatterbrained over little things like checking the petrol gauge. It was one of her many endearing features.

She parked up, got a can out of the back and set off in search of a 24-hour garage. She was slightly built and timid and would not have been looking forward to the walk so late at night. She was only out at all because she had taken a job at a pub in Bebington to make some extra cash before her forthcoming wedding.

If she had noticed Sullivan following her she would have been very scared. If he had leaped out of the shadows at her she would have been rigid with fear. Either way she would have been no match for Sullivan, the victim, the loser, driven by demons no one will ever comprehend.

In a confession that he later retracted he said he stopped Diane to ask her the time and then exploded with a sudden desire to kill. But Sullivan did much more than that. Her body was to tell a story of terrible frenzy. This was no mere murder.

Everyone who saw what he had done to her was shaken. Police, doctors, nurses – and me. There are limits and this was far beyond them.

It was at 3.50 p.m. on Saturday, 2 August that I was taken by senior police officers with forensic scientist Graham Jackson, from the laboratory at Chorley, Lancashire, to an alleyway off Borough Road. I was shown the body of a young female lying face upwards, unclothed except for some garments around the neck. Rigor mortis was fully developed. Clearly, she had been dead for some hours.

It took more than an hour to carry out a detailed forensic examination of the site with the body *in situ*. She was then taken to the mortuary at Arrowe Park Hospital, Birkenhead, where I began my preliminary examination at 5.30 p.m.

Diane measured five feet, six inches tall. We noticed how slim she was.

The clothing around the neck was seen to consist of a bra and white T-shirt with green dots. The T-shirt was bloodstained and the right strap of the bra was undone. They were wrapped only loosely around the neck. A broken metal necklace was found and removed. She was wearing a diamond engagement ring.

The body was cleaned and an examination was made by a forensic odontologist. He had been called in by the police because of the bite marks.

When he had finished photographing and noting every detail of the bites I recommenced my post-mortem examination at 7.35 p.m.

There were three lacerations to Diane's forehead. The first, above the right eyebrow, half an inch long and three quarters of an inch in width, exposed the bone beneath. The second, a diagonal wound one and a half inches long was in the midline or centre of the forehead. The third was one and a quarter inches long and above the left eyebrow.

There was bruising around both eyes with petechial haemorrhages in the conjunctiva and cuts to both upper eyelids. Her nose was broken.

The right side of the chin showed bruising with numerous lacerations. A deep laceration, one inch long over the lower jaw, exposed the bone beneath. The mouth was distorted due to fractures of both the upper and lower jaws on the right side. The impact had also loosened the teeth.

There was a bruise on the left side of the neck and a haemorrhagic mark three inches by one across the larynx with linear abrasions on the right side of the neck.

Both breasts showed abrasions and circulatory bruises consistent with biting. The right nipple had been mutilated and the left nipple was missing. We found the left nipple in her umbilicus (navel).

Assuming it had not simply become lodged there by accident but had been placed there by hand, it was, while undeniably gruesome, nevertheless a peculiarly precise and delicate moment of order during what would have been a wild and frenetic sequence of events.

[Two months later I returned to the hospital to watch a second post-mortem being performed on behalf of the defence lawyers. On that occasion Mr Jackson, the scientist, showed me a piece of tissue that had been found subsequently in the alleyway where Diane had been killed. It was the other nipple.]

Both arms showed small, brown abrasions and there was bruising on the back middle, third and little fingers of the left hand.

The external genitalia showed bruising with two ragged lacerations in the anterior area, the first one inch long and the second half an inch long, both above the vaginal orifice. A further laceration was seen below the vaginal orifice. There was an abrasion on the inner aspect of the right thigh.

Both knees were bruised and had scrape marks. There were brown abrasions on the back of the right shoulder and further superficial abrasions over the lower abdomen.

Cause of Death

A scrape on the back of the right thigh and abrasions on the back of the right lower leg and at the right ankle were consistent with Diane having been heaved across the ground by her shoulders, with her feet dragging behind.

Internally the skull was fractured on each side and over the vault with severe comminution of the anterior cranial fossa. In other words, she had been hit repeatedly and with extreme force across the head and her skull had been crushed like an eggshell at breakfast. The brain showed haemorrhage over the surface, with bruising of the cortex in the temporal areas.

There was bruising in the neck on each side of the larynx, which was oedematous (swollen), and extensive fractures of the thyroid cartilage. The trachea and bronchi contained inhaled blood, which was also present in the lungs. The mouth contained blood and showed fractures of the right upper and lower jaws, bruising and loose teeth.

I concluded that Diane had suffered four or five heavy blows to the head and face with a blunt instrument. She had also sustained a heavy blow across the larynx and to the external genitalia, also with a blunt instrument. I confirmed that the injuries to the breasts were consistent with biting.

She had died of a cerebral haemorrhage.

The savagery of the killing shocked Merseyside and led to the biggest – to that date – murder hunt in the city's history. But for weeks the police got nowhere.

Amazingly, no one had seen or heard anything while this brutal and sustained attack was going on. The severity of the injuries left little doubt that Diane would have died very quickly once the blows rained down, but she was then dragged backwards and stripped almost naked. This takes at least a couple of minutes with an unhelpful body and that is a long time in a street murder.

Diane's jeans, panties, green high-heeled shoes and handbag were not found at the murder scene. Police assumed, rightly, that they had been taken by the killer. Sullivan, who must have been covered in blood, took them home and hid them before washing and climbing into bed with his common-law wife.

Two weeks on the items were found burned on Bidston Hill a little way out of the town. They revealed nothing useful in themselves but a witness recalled seeing a man whom he knew vaguely behaving oddly on the hill. The man, he told detectives, was called Peter, had a long nose and tattooed arms – and liked darts.

On 22 September a policeman in plain clothes walked into a pub in Birkenhead and got talking to Peter Sullivan. They chatted about darts and the officer noted the man's pointed nose and his forearm tattoos.

Three days later, after Sullivan's home had been searched, I was shown a crowbar and asked whether it could have been used as the murder weapon in this case. I said it could. The majority of the injuries could have been caused by the stem; the claw end could have caused the injury to the right side of the forehead and the jemmy end could have caused two or three of the injuries on the right side of the lower jaw.

Sullivan pleaded not guilty. The jury decided he was a liar as well as a loser.

The clinching evidence was that of the odontologist who told the jury that the bite marks on Diane's body matched the accused man's teeth perfectly. They were as unique as a fingerprint and just as damning.

As with 'Beast of the Night' Trevor Joseph Hardy, the Press was quick to give Diane Sindall's killer a nickname. 'The Wolfman' was one, 'The Mersey Ripper' another.

This worthless individual deserved nothing so romantic or dramatic.

Stuart Brownhill could have killed three people in less than twenty-four hours. Some believe, had he succeeded, he might have had the inclination to kill a few more. Certainly he had all the attributes of a serial killer: anger, low self-esteem, natural brutality and a callous disregard for anyone but himself. In short, he was a nasty piece of work.

As it was he murdered just one person, a fun-loving mother called Lynne Taylor who had the bad luck to meet him while she was out on the town.

About two a.m. on Thursday, 30 August 1984, a couple got into a taxi outside Fritters nightclub in Oldham. The driver remembered that during the journey the man briefly got out of the cab and shouted at someone in a house.

The woman turned to the cabbie and said, with a chuckle: 'What have I got myself into?' The man then climbed back in and the taxi took them to Number 12, Monmouth Street in the Werneth area of the town.

The driver heard the man ask the woman if he could come in for a cup of tea and, reluctantly, she said that he could. It was a considerable error of judgement on her part.

At breakfast-time passers-by on their way to work noticed that the front windows of the terraced house were blackened and there was a slight smell of burning.

There was no reply to their knocks on the door so a neighbour called the police who broke in. Clouds of drifting smoke from the fire that had burned itself out made it difficult to see. But Lynne Taylor was quickly spotted, lying on her back, obviously dead, on the floor in the centre of the living room.

The neighbour ran upstairs to the back bedroom where she found Lynne's eleven-year-old son, Geoffrey. He was sleeping peacefully, unharmed and completely unaware of the horrors of the previous few hours or that he had nearly been burned to death. The neighbour took him out the back way.

I arrived at 1.16 p.m. I have to be precise about my timings because I am often asked to establish the time of death. It was a small room with a TV in one corner on a stand and a gas fire on the wall. A circular shag-pile rug about five feet in diameter was in front of the fire, over the patterned fitted carpet. There was a settee and matching armchair but the cushion from the settee had been removed and placed on the floor.

Lynne Taylor, thirty-one years old, was lying on the cushion, face up in a spread-eagle position, her legs and arms splayed. Her short red dress and bra had been pushed up to her neck, exposing her breasts. She was wearing a suspender belt and stockings but her knickers had been pulled down to the stocking tops. Protruding from the vagina was a wooden rolling pin. It rested on the stretched band of her knickers.

Below the legs the cushion was severely burned. Lynne's left thigh was burned and there was extensive smoke-staining of the entire body and of the room.

The doors to the room were sealed and the fire had

burned only a short period, dying down as the oxygen level in the room dropped.

Three hours later, at Oldham mortuary, Mrs Taylor was measured at five feet, four inches in height and weighed just over nine stone.

Petechial (pinprick) haemorrhages were present in both eyes, with larger haemorrhages at the angles of each eye. The upper lip was bruised and the lower lip bruised and lacerated. The left ear lobe was lacerated and missing an earring. There was an abrasion one inch long by half an inch wide on the left side of the chin.

Three silver necklaces were around the neck and there was bruising across the front of the neck, with small abrasions on the left side. Just below the left collarbone there was a bruise roughly circular in shape and about three-quarters of an inch in diameter. There were three bruises on the inside of the left upper arm over a three-inch-by-one-inch area. The right arm showed an area of bruising above the elbow over a slightly smaller area. These were consistent with the application of force by fingers, perhaps when dragging a person backwards by the upper arms.

The right thigh showed an area of burning ten inches long that extended around the back of the leg.

The rolling pin was removed from the vagina. Four inches had been inserted and it was bloodstained. It was removed with difficulty.

The scalp showed numerous petechial haemorrhages on the internal surface with an area of bruising in the left parietal area. The brain was healthy.

There was no evidence of inhaled fumes and the level of carbon monoxide in the blood was only eight per cent, showing that she was dead before the fire started.

The larynx was intact but there were petechial haemorrhages at the base of the epiglottis and on the surface of the lungs, which were congested.

Lynne Taylor had died, I concluded, from asphyxia caused by pressure to the neck. The rolling pin and the fire, mercifully, both happened later.

The taxi driver's description of the man now wanted for murder was circulated. The following evening a policeman was called to a violent dispute between a couple where the woman claimed that the man had threatened to kill her.

With hindsight it appears that she had good reason to be worried. The officer recognized similarities with the description of the murder suspect and arrested twenty-eight-year-old Stuart Brownhill. The killer had only been released from prison nine days earlier.

It was not long before he confessed to the murder. But first he told a series of lies about his victim, alleging that she had taunted him after agreeing to have sex.

Eventually Brownhill told the truth: Lynne hadn't wanted him and he had strangled her after attempting to rape her.

He also admitted that he knew the boy was asleep upstairs when he set the fire. 'I just wanted to get rid of the evidence,' he told police.

Brownhill pleaded guilty to murder and arson with intent to endanger life. He was sentenced to life imprisonment by a judge at Manchester Crown Court.

But before that, shortly after his arrest, he staged a hunger strike while being held on remand. When questioned about the reasons for the self-imposed fast, his lawyer told bemused magistrates: 'He doesn't see any future for himself.'

Let's hope he was right.

For some odd reason sex crimes and fire seem to have an affinity. When an attempt is made to burn away evidence following a murder one usually finds the action has a sexual association.

I can offer no good reason for this.

Such was the case with Winifred Smith, an unfortunate spinster of forty-seven years who had a flat in Rusland Court, Blackley, Manchester.

When I got there at 12.25 p.m. on Monday, 23 March 1987, the fire had not been long out and the settee was still smouldering. The body had been at the side of the settee but was now outside the front door to the flat after a rescue attempt.

I pronounced life extinct – that's always a good precaution if someone hasn't checked first – and took a preliminary look.

There was extensive smoke-staining to the back of the body and ligatures were obvious around the mouth and neck.

Winifred Smith was just five feet tall and weighed a mere seven stone. Her clothes consisted of a blue shirt, pink knickers and white bra, which were all removed and bagged prior to the examination.

There were several abrasions and bruises on the forehead, the bridge of the nose, the right cheek and the left upper lip. The eyelids of the left eye were bruised and both eyes were congested.

Across the mouth were three loops of stocking material, tightly applied, which passed across the head leaving a groove half an inch wide along where there were haemorrhagic marks. Knots had been tied in the material and were present on the left side of the neck and at the back.

There was smoke-staining on the front of the right forearm, back of the left forearm, both buttocks, the backs of the left thigh, the right leg and both hands.

Internally, the trachea and bronchi contained frothy and bloodstained fluid. The larynx showed slight bruising and the superior horn on each side was fractured. The lungs were congested with scanty petechial haemorrhages on the pleural surface.

Miss Smith had been strangled with her own stockings by someone who had also beaten her severely around the face and then started a fire underneath her body.

The reason twenty-three-year-old local man David Hughes gave for killing her after he pleaded guilty to the crime was that she might have given him Aids after they had sex.

I was asked whether or not I had carried out an Aids test on the dead woman's body.

I had. She did not have the virus.

If Mr Hughes was telling the truth he had made a grave mistake.

Father-of-two Edward Fleming was on his best behaviour the night there was a fire at a neighbour's flat.

Firemen had raced to Askam Close, Blackburn late on a Friday in June 1987 after reports that someone might be trapped in their home. Tragically it was true. When they arrived, too late, they found the living room well alight and the body of a young woman lying by the side of a chair.

It wasn't exactly an inferno but she was quite badly burned and, as detailed elsewhere in these chapters, all you need is to inhale some of those fumes and you've had it. She was pulled clear straight away and the firemen tried resuscitation techniques. But it was obviously in vain. The fire was extinguished quickly. It was sad but routine.

Marie Ashton was only nineteen years old, a barmaid at a club called the Peppermint Place in Blackburn. For policemen, ambulance crews, pathologists and firemen, it is always worse when the victim is young. It always has that much more of an emotional effect.

Mr Fleming, thirty-four, with his wife expecting their third child, was soon out with the tea and sympathy, literally. He made the firemen cups of tea while they waited for formalities to be carried out after they had extinguished the blaze.

The entire street came out, as you might expect with all the noise and hullabaloo. It was a terrible shame for Marie, everyone agreed. Must have been a cigarette.

She was taken to the mortuary at the town's Queen's Park Hospital and placed in a fridge until the morning. The following day, quite early, the mortuary attendant arrived at work, checked the log, and set about his tasks. The first was to clean up the body of an unfortunate young woman killed in a fire.

He started at the head and had only travelled down a few inches when he stopped in his tracks. An experienced man, he knew bodies could contort and twist into odd positions in death, he knew fires could do terrible things, and he knew never to draw instant conclusions. But he also knew that fires don't strangle people. There was a distinctive mark on the girl's neck that needed looking at.

I got the call that morning and arrived at the hospital shortly after ten a.m. At eleven a.m., at the request of the coroner for Blackburn, I began the examination.

Marie Ashton was just over five feet, three inches tall and had blistering on the nose, on each cheek, and on the lobe of the right ear. The eyes were swollen and haemorrhagic. The tongue was protruding through the teeth.

The front of the body showed extensive red burns with brown staining and blackening of both arms and hands. There was a blue bruise two inches in diameter on the left upper arm. The back showed areas of burning. Both legs were extensively charred, the skin had split and exposed the muscles underneath.

The neck showed blistering on the right side and there was a linear mark, four inches long, at the level of the larynx on the front left side. The back of the neck had a linear haemorrhagic mark in continuity with the mark on the front.

Burned clothing had been removed but there were the remains of a skirt and a white striped blouse. Marie also still had her knickers.

Internally, the scalp showed a bruise on the frontal area with small petechial haemorrhages. There was slight bruising of the strap muscles on the left side of the neck. The larynx was intact but there were petechial haemorrhages in the epiglottis and mucosa of the larynx.

The trachea and bronchi were healthy but they showed no sign of the smoke that one might expect with someone who had died in a fire. The lungs were congested and had petechial haemorrhages on the surface but no sign of inhaled fumes.

The tip of the tongue showed teeth marks, probably her own. The toxicology tests found no significant trace of carbon monoxide.

I felt the findings were classically consistent with Marie having been strangled with a ligature.

Furthermore, she had died before the fire had started. It had only damaged the outside of her body, she had breathed none of it in.

It didn't take the police long. They searched Marie's flat and found a set of keys belonging to Fleming who was a bouncer at the Peppermint Place and had come home with her on the Friday night.

He soon admitted his part. Rather than him going straight home, they had gone instead back to her flat and had begun making love. But he had been drinking too much and couldn't manage it. He claimed she burst out laughing and made a comment about what his wife would say if she knew about what they were up to – or not, as the case might be.

With the twisted logic typical of violent men, Fleming told the court that one of the reasons he had used force was that he had been worried his wife might lose their child if Marie spilled the beans about their secrets.

He put a piece of cord around Marie's neck, intending, he said, to frighten her into answering his questions about what she intended to do. He heard a noise 'like a gargle' and she fell forward. When he realized she was dead he panicked, started the fire and went home. Little wonder he was sufficiently awake to be able to offer the firemen cups of tea shortly afterwards.

Fleming pleaded guilty to manslaughter. But the jury found him guilty of murder and he got life.

Sex was almost certainly not the motive, however, for the murder of 'Chattie' Ann Chadderton, whose burned body was found in the early spring of 1979 at the second-hand clothing shop she ran from what was little more than a wooden shack in Wilshaw Lane, Ashton-Under-Lyne.

I was shown the remains of the well-liked fifty-eight-year-old lying face downwards amongst the charred remains of clothing.

She was not a big woman by any means, at just five feet, one inch in height. Of course, it makes sense that so many victims of violence are small when you consider that the vast majority of people who commit acts of violence are weak, fearful and inadequate people who can find no other way to cope with adversity.

Mrs Chadderton had severe burns to her right upper arm, the middle of the trunk, the front of the thighs, the left hand, the buttocks, and the back of the right leg, with smoke-staining on the right hand and around the face.

But, again, the fire hadn't killed her. 'Chattie Annie', a mumsy, cheery character with a good word for everyone, had been stabbed forty-one times.

Of the penetrative wounds, seventeen were into the left side of her chest through the back, one into the right side and another to the right side of the lower abdomen. They were caused by an instrument which had both a sharp edge and a blunt edge. There were a further nineteen wounds that were superficial, caused most likely by a blunt blade.

Three linear bruises on the neck were consistent with

finger pressure. These, with petechial haemorrhages to the lower neck and in the conjunctiva of both eyes, suggested an attempt at manual strangulation.

Internally, the larynx showed bruising, with fractures of the superior horns of the thyroid cartilage on each side. The trachea and bronchi contained blood. The lungs contained inhaled blood and the left upper lobe had five stab wounds. The left pleural cavity contained about a pint of blood and blood clot. The chest wall showed stab wounds adjacent to the third, fifth, sixth, seventh and eighth ribs close to the spine on the left side.

Death resulted from haemorrhage and shock caused by both the stabbing and the manual strangulation. This was overkill.

Later I was shown a pair of scissors and a knife blade bearing the legend 'Stainless Steel Japan'. I agreed that the knife would have been capable of causing the superficial wounds while the scissors could have caused the penetrative wounds.

They had been taken from an individual who had confessed to the killing, sixteen-year-old Wayne Millin, one of Chattie Annie's regulars.

He said he had gone into the shop to return a pair of trousers he had bought for £1.50 that did not fit. While there he attacked her in a ferocious fashion before starting three fires. He left with the cash float, estimated at between £50 and £100.

Before the murder the teenager had cashed a cheque from his father's chequebook for £12. Shortly after the killing he repaid the debt.

The boy himself never offered a reasonable explanation for his appalling act. But if Mrs Chadderton died because he was scared about nicking £12 from his dad then his priorities were outrageously out of phase. But then, that is so often the case.

Psychiatrists could find no sign of mental illness in Millin and because of his age he was sentenced to be 'detained during her Majesty's Pleasure'.

13

Cold and Steel

The murder that probably gave me the most satisfaction was that of Norman Clarke.

He died just two hours into the year 1991 and was found collapsed in the street by a bunch of New Year revellers on their way to another party.

As it happened, that year was to be a bumper year for murders in Greater Manchester. The death toll had started both early and in a rush with fatalities from natural causes too.

The holiday period meant that there were fewer pathologists around than usual. The cases were flooding in so I was asked to fill in at the Manchester mortuary on my day off.

Norman, recently retired from his job as a hospital porter at Stepping Hill Hospital, Stockport, was sixty-three years old, a widower and not a robust man. Outwardly there was nothing unduly worrying about the case and it looked like a simple, tragic collapse.

He still had his wallet and watch and that seemed to rule out any suspicions about it being a robbery gone wrong. Further, he was still wearing his glasses, thus removing, surely, any ideas that he had been involved in a violent struggle. Sadly but simply, he'd just gone down like a sack of potatoes and probably never knew it was happening. If you could pick a way to go, that would be many people's first choice.

This was going to be routine. I was looking at a heart attack, a brain haemorrhage, something straightforward, something common. Natural causes.

Norman's body had been discovered in Princess Road, Moss Side, a direct route by which he could make his way home on foot from where he'd seen in the New Year. Other than the obvious scratches and scrapes associated with falling hard in the street there was no reason to call the death suspicious. Nothing, that was until I looked behind his ear.

Hidden by his hair and the curve of the ear flap was a small cut that had seeped hardly any blood but was quite new. I peeled away the skin and checked the skull. A neat hole no more than four millimetres in diameter – the width of a large nail – had penetrated the thinnest part of the bone, close to the temple.

An internal examination showed that, while thin, the instrument was quite long and had penetrated four inches into Norman Clarke's brain. He had died instantly.

I cried murder and called in the police. But I still cannot fully comprehend the reaction I got.

While I was immediately certain that we were dealing with an unlawful killing, it would be fair to admit that there was nothing spectacular or overly complex about this death. Quite the reverse, in fact. Indeed, it was so *un*spectacular that it seemed that everyone who should have been running around getting excited almost dismissed it.

At first the senior detectives – perhaps themselves short of men over the holiday – were reluctant even to call it a murder. But the thing about murder investigations is that the faster they get under way the better chance they have of success. Witnesses are still around, their memories are fresh. Information is easier to come by.

This inquiry really didn't get into full swing for about three days. Even after I'd shown the wound to the man in charge, Detective Superintendent Ron Gaffey, he took some convincing.

The police argument was that the victim might have tripped and banged his head on something sharp on the way down. Maybe, they suggested, optimistically, it was an accident.

Much to their disappointment I insisted that despite the fact there was no apparent motive, no weapon and no witnesses, this was nevertheless a murder and they had to start looking for a killer. The further bad news for them was that they had absolutely nothing to go on.

Mr Clarke was a teetotal solitary individual, very quiet, with few friends and no enemies. On the night he died he had been in the Big Western pub in Moss Side, Manchester, where up to 400 people were enjoying themselves. After five days a thirty-man murder squad had traced just forty. It was that kind of pub.

Late on, a barmaid recalled, Clarke fell asleep in a chair, then woke up, was served with an orange juice and left, alone, at around two a.m. He never made it even halfway home to West Didsbury and no one could produce a good reason why.

Inevitably, the police inquiry was eventually wound down. Without any leads the best detective in the world is useless.

At the inquest into the death the Manchester coroner, Leonard Gorodkin, said that while Mr Clarke did not look like he had been attacked, the injury was unlikely to have been due to an accident. While having no information about who did it or how it happened, he said he accepted my professional opinion that death had been caused by a third party. As a consequence, he recorded a verdict of unlawful killing.

I suggested then that the sort of weapon capable of causing such an injury would be something like a butcher's skewer, that is, something hard, long and thin. Being pointed at the end would have helped, too.

After that hearing Mr Clarke's brother, while obviously disappointed that the truth was still unknown, said he thought the police had done all they could. He was, he said, happy with the verdict.

In most cases that would have been it. An ordinary man with few connections dies and not too many people care. The system has a stab at establishing the truth but, as the detail of what happened doesn't fit the usual pigeon-holes, the system fails. End of story.

Except, out of the blue, eighteen months later, a twenty-four-year-old man from Beswick, an area a couple of miles from where Mr Clarke died, confessed, apparently because his conscience got to him.

It wasn't a skewer or a nail, explained Michael Ryan. It was a screwdriver. He had stopped a hunched, bespectacled figure in the street and asked him for a light. Norman Clarke, perhaps startled or afraid, had pushed the younger man away.

Ryan admitted he struck out, intending to hit the older man's arm. But, by what Ryan's defence counsel later described as 'the greatest ill chance', the blow missed its target and followed through to the side of Clarke's head.

That Ryan also happened to have a screwdriver in his hand was, naturally, another matter for consideration by the court. But it had to be accepted that, at that time of night in most inner cities and most certainly in Manchester, it was far from unusual for young men to carry 'protection'. To keep a screwdriver hidden in your pocket would be considered no more than a sensible precaution to the street-wise.

The prosecution, having no case other than the man's own confession, accepted his plea of not guilty to murder but guilty to manslaughter.

The judge at Liverpool Crown Court had to weigh two important matters in deciding punishment. In the defendant's favour was the fact that this was a sincerely remorseful man who had, through his voluntary confession, brought the prosecution wholly upon himself. Against him was his own damning evidence that he had used a screwdriver, without warning and without provocation, on a frail sixty-three-year-old man making his way peacefully home early on New Year's Day.

The judge sentenced Ryan to six years.

Thinking about it, I was probably the only person to get any satisfaction whatsoever out of that particular tragedy.

Just down the road from where Mr Clarke fell was possibly the unluckiest nightclub in Manchester. The Nile Club never pretended to be the Ritz – not even the Ritz in Whitworth Street, famous for its bouncy dance floor and 1970s nights.

The clientele of the Nile didn't expect too much in the way of plush soft furnishings, fine wines and deferential service from discreet waitresses – although discretion was rarely a bad idea.

It was next door to the New Reno Club, the two establishments sharing a great deal of available space on three floors of a semi-derelict Victorian red-brick building on Princess Road that was for many years somewhat overshadowed by a brewery and has since been flattened.

Inside, the large main room had a central area for dancing, which was surrounded by basic tables and chairs, and most of the floor area was covered in old lino with an orange-and-yellow square pattern. Where it wasn't faded and ripped, the wallpaper was stained with damp and there was a pervading musty smell in the air from old beer bottles, cigarettes and sweat. In short, it was a dump.

But it was a popular dump.

It was run very much on a club basis where only regulars or those whom regulars chose to invite would be welcome. And that way people felt more relaxed, at ease – safe. There was regular gambling – sometimes for quite high stakes – and it was a place where deals could be done, meetings held, business conducted.

Also, importantly, before the licensing laws were relaxed in the rest of Britain they were already very relaxed at the Nile. It was, in many ways, ahead of its time.

Unfortunately, the club also had a tendency to get blood-stained – on two occasions, to my certain knowledge, with fatal consequences.

In 1975 the place was owned – or at least run – by a forty-eight-year-old father of four, very active and popular in the local community, who revelled in the splendid name of Sunday 'Sunny' Nwagbara. He was well built though not a big man – five feet, eight inches tall and eleven stone, eight pounds in weight – but he was known as a good conciliator and an accomplished negotiator in many spheres. In his line of business, he had to be.

When I met him on 25 May 1975, he was naked, dead and in my mortuary in Manchester.

There were fresh abrasions on both his legs but neither was of any great significance. His problems lay at the other end of his body. There was extensive bruising of the scalp in the occipital area (back of the head) and a comminuted fracture of the occipital bone that was linear across the base of the skull with radiating fractures from each end.

The surface of the brain showed haemorrhage with contrecoup bruising on the front and temporal lobes. There was slight softening of the brain substance in the occipital area. The trachea and bronchi contained a bloodstained, watery exudate and the lungs were oedematous.

Sunny had died from a brain haemorrhage caused by a powerful blow to the back of his head. A tough man, he survived for two hours after being struck but would have remained unconscious and would have known very little, if anything, about it.

He had been hit at nine o'clock in the morning at the conclusion of the Nile's nocturnal activities – which tended to last somewhat longer than in most clubs.

The man who had hit him, thirty-six-year-old Gerald Foster, was a gambler who admitted in court to having lost 'thousands of pounds' playing poker. By this stage he had clearly realized that gambling is a mug's game. But it would have been better all round if he had learned his lesson earlier.

When Foster walked into the Nile he was carrying £600 and looking for a game. When he left he was broke and looking for a reason.

What had happened in the intervening period was a matter of disagreement during the murder trial. Foster claimed he was winning at cards when another player offered him a cigar. It was drugged and after a few puffs he passed out to wake up with all his cash gone. Unable to do anything about it but angry at being robbed, he asked for enough money to pay for a taxi to a friend's house but was told in no uncertain terms to be on his way.

Sunny and another man who was carrying a briefcase containing the night's takings were moving Foster off the premises, he insisted, when the second man swung at him with the case. He explained how he grabbed an iron bar, which was on the floor, and lashed out to protect himself. The blow missed its intended target and hit Sunny on the head. Foster then grabbed the bag, which he thought at the time contained his stolen money, and fled.

The prosecution, on the other hand, thought the cigar story was, as it were, so much smoke. They maintained that Foster had lost his money and in frustration had felled the club owner and stolen the cash to make up his losses.

The jury was less sure about the way the verdict should go than I was. Perhaps they had come across more spiked cigars than I had. They decided Foster was guilty of manslaughter, not murder.

The judge, however, seemed to agree with me. Foster literally staggered in the dock with shock when he heard Mr Justice Jupp sentence him to fifteen years – much longer than he could reasonably have expected for a conviction on the lesser charge.

Now, when a case begins the judge knows a heck of a lot more than the jury. In most cases he will have his own ideas about what the verdict should be. But, of course, he must keep these to himself and allow the twelve chosen men and women to make up their own minds, no matter how feeble or criminally inclined those minds might be.

The verdict of the jury in this case was manslaughter, not murder, and the judge had to sentence Foster according to their findings.

A few days after the case Mr Justice Jupp ordered Foster to be brought back before him. The killer must have feared that his tormentor was about to don the black cap and finish the job. But the learned judge instead informed the surprised man: 'I have reconsidered your case and, to match the jury's verdict of manslaughter, I have reduced your sentence to ten years.'

An even more generous judgement was made on the man responsible for my second acquaintance with the Nile, which also involved my first and only visit to the establishment.

When I arrived a policeman was standing guard outside the door and I was invited to go up the steps and into the main room. Cecil 'Hovis' Brown, a well-built forty-four-year-old black man with a shaven head, was lying face up on the bloodstained lino floor in a corner close to an exit door.

The front of his trousers was heavily stained with blood and his bloodstained blue pullover had been rolled up to reveal his chest. There were two clear puncture wounds on the left side of his chest, close to the mid-line, and a further injury to his nose. Blood was spattered over a nearby chair and table and in several other areas in the room as far as twenty feet from the body.

At the mortuary I was able to establish that the injuries were stab wounds. The first was half an inch long and cut through the left side of the nose into the nasal cavity. On the chest the wounds were both horizontal, about one inch from the mid-line and separated from each other by about an inch. The higher wound was three-quarters of an inch long and the lower wound one and a half inches long. They had entered above and below the fourth rib, damaging the upper and lower borders of the rib cartilage on the way, and had penetrated to a depth of about six inches. The direction of the blow was inwards and across to the right side.

Internally the lungs showed slight congestion, the right pleural cavity was healthy but the left contained about two pints of blood. The heart was enlarged but this was due to hypertrophy of the left ventricle, itself probably caused by high blood pressure and not connected with the injuries sustained. The pericardium was bruised and the pericardial sac contained blood clot.

The front of the heart showed two parallel wounds corresponding to the wounds in the chest. These had both entered the anterior (front) wall of the right ventricle, penetrated the septum and entered the left ventricle. The upper wound emerged through the posterior (rear) wall of the heart.

Had the upper wound been marginally lower and the lower wound marginally higher both would have struck the rib and might have been deflected to relative safety or even prevented from penetrating to any significant degree at all. As it was they both sliced through easily, missed the bone, and speared the heart of Cecil 'Hovis' Brown. The lower, deeper wound went all the way through and came out the other side. Even if an ambulance had been waiting outside the front door of the club with its engine running, Hovis would never have completed the mile-long journey to

Manchester Royal Infirmary alive.

He had been killed by Warren Adams, aged fifty, a friend he had known for years who had arrived at the Nile carrying a black-handled Skyline kitchen knife with a blade a little under six inches long and a little more than one inch wide at its broadest point. At his trial the accused man insisted the instrument of death was on his person for no other reason than to allow him to carry out a little temporary repair work on a broken window.

When they met at the Nile they had a row about Mr Adams's girlfriend who had been Mr Brown's girlfriend. As Hovis moved forward, so did the knife. Twice. It is likely that the third wound, to his nose, happened as he fell, something he would have done pretty much straight away.

Mr Adams pleaded not guilty to murder, claiming self-defence. Hovis, he said, had thrown a bottle at him and then rushed towards him and grabbed his jacket lapels. It was at this point, he told the jury at Manchester Crown Court, that he reached into his pocket and found the knife. He held it in front of him to frighten his furious friend – but Hovis kept coming.

Crucial to the defence was the manner in which the knife was being held. Mr Adams said he was holding it in his right hand with the palm facing upwards. While this is just as dangerous as any other method of holding a knife, it is a much less aggressive stance than, say, holding it above one's head with the knuckles above the blade.

My findings and those of a second pathologist called by the defence were that the injuries were consistent with what Adams was saying about the attack. The jury, satisfied he was telling the truth about the physics of the stabbing, chose also to believe his statement that his intention was never to harm Hovis, merely to scare him. They acquitted him of murder and he walked free.

While the knife – be it flick, lock, hunting, fishing, kitchen, bread or pen – is probably the most favoured murder weapon because of its ease of handling and deadly capability, any number of pointed instruments have been known to cause terminal damage.

Mr Clarke, mentioned earlier in this chapter, died from a blow through his brain with a screwdriver. The screwdriver, stiff and sharp, was perfect for that task. Paradoxically, had the killer been better armed, Mr Clarke might have survived and Ryan would not have gone to jail. Some slim-bladed knives might have failed to break through the bones of the skull and caused little more than superficial damage to the scalp.

Saadat Khan, forty-seven, from Burnley, died after becoming involved in a street fracas in the summer of 1984. I was asked to examine his body at Burnley public mortuary.

He had a laceration of the right nostril that extended on to the upper lip and into the mouth. It could have been caused by any number of sharp instruments.

On the left side of the chest was a circular wound, very neat, slightly elliptical and three-quarters of an inch in diameter. Internally it passed upwards and inwards for about five inches. There were also small abrasions on the front of both knees and the back of the little finger.

While the right pleural cavity was healthy, the left contained about three and a half pints of blood and blood clot. The wound in the chest wall had entered the chest cavity between the sixth and seventh ribs and passed over the left lobe of the diaphragm to enter the apex of the heart. A circular wound half an inch in diameter was present and extended into the internal chamber of the left ventricle, through the interventricular septum and into the right ventricle. It came to a stop as it hit the opposite wall just below the pulmonary valve.

Mr Khan had died from haemorrhage caused by a penetrating wound to the chest, a wound that had pierced his heart.

It was the sort of wound, though a little too wide, that might be caused by the accurate thrust by a swordsman of a rapier.

Later, I was shown a number of potential weapons labelled one to ten. I decided that the injury could have been caused by either weapon eight or weapon nine.

It turned out to be weapon eight, the shaft of a golf club – a No. 3 wood, I think.

A neighbour, Younis Khan, pleaded guilty to manslaughter, arguing that he had never intended to kill his namesake. Clearly the judge believed him because he considered the time the man had spent in custody awaiting trial, sentenced him to that period of imprisonment, and set him free.

Clovis O'Neil Craig died from a single blow with a machete – but in genuinely million-to-one circumstances.

That same summer he was working at his garage, the Nottingham Motor Engineering company, in Johnson Street, Old Trafford, Manchester, when a friend arrived, a very irate friend. Carlton Lyons was usually a mild-mannered teacher but he was also a former captain of the England amateur boxing team, so he was not someone to

247

mess with.

On this occasion, though, his mild manner had given way to fury and, although they were usually pals, Clovis and Carlton rowed loudly over a £90 debt. To add insult to injury, Clovis then produced the money Carlton thought should be coming to him and promptly handed it over to someone else.

Enraged, but still in moderate control, the boxer from Stockport who had fought for his country against Scotland and Holland in the 1970s went back to his car and produced a large ornamental Japanese sword.

Standing several feet away, far out of reach, Lyons assumed a martial arts fighting stance and swung the blade back over his shoulder before bringing it down with force.

When I arrived at the garage Clovis Craig was lying on his right side, still in his overalls, white sweater and trousers.

At the mortuary at Park Hospital, Davyhulme, we examined Craig's clothing and found a one-inch cut on the front of the sweater which was directly over a wound in the chest. There was a transverse laceration in the midline, just below the notch of the sternum and just under one and a quarter inches long. It travelled towards the back and slightly to the right.

The lungs were collapsed and there was a laceration that passed through the right upper lobe and then continued to travel for just under seven inches into the body to pierce the second rib at the back about one inch from the midline on the right side. The pleural cavities contained four pints of blood and there was a laceration in the arch of the aorta, the main blood vessel coming out of the heart.

In short, a single stabbing motion had sent the blade

through the breastbone, sliced a fatal wound in the aorta, continued cutting through the right lung and embedded itself in the back of the ribcage. Mr Craig had bled to death very quickly.

I was shown a blade twenty inches long and one and a quarter inches wide, which curved to a point and had blood staining approximately seven inches from the tip. I agreed the injury could have been caused by this blade. It had no handle.

In the moment when Carlton Lyons had swung in anger, the blade had snapped off from the hilt. It could have flown anywhere – but it flew straight at Carlton's friend. It could have struck him a glancing blow with the flat side or missed altogether, but it didn't. Even with penetration the chances were that it would not cause life-threatening injuries. But it did.

Fate took the blade at the worst possible angle between Clovis Craig's ribs, into the most delicate part of the chest, and severed a main vein.

Lyons told police when they arrived at the scene: 'I don't know what happened. He was miles away.'

Lyons was obviously devastated by what he had done. Mr Justice Cantley took pity on him and told him: 'I have never heard of anything like this before.' The judge sentenced him to two years for manslaughter. As a further act of compassion he suspended sixteen months of the sentence, allowing the killer to walk free out of the court.

The boxer was clearly no danger to anyone any more.

On his way home on the top deck of a bus one cold December night a passenger was half asleep, resting his head on the side of the window but unable to settle because it kept bumping him awake. As his eyes opened reluctantly for the umpteenth time he saw a strange vision through the leafless branches of the trees.

It was the shape of a man, a naked man, and around him were dotted, in a near-perfect circle a number of objects that reflected the moonlight. It was like a watch face. The bus bumped again and, as the passenger blinked, the vision vanished.

He shook his head, decided it was a ridiculous notion and tried to forget about it. A few days later, when nothing had appeared in the papers, on TV or local radio, he contacted the Cheshire police. It was Christmas Eve.

They went out to a wooded area, just outside Crewe, discovered he had not been dreaming and called me.

Now, while most people resent working over Christmas I have become resigned to it. Christmas is a time when a lot of people die: a time of bad weather, of excessive drinking, of great emotions and deep depressions. We pathologists expect to be busy at Christmas.

This was to be one of my last jobs in that part of the world, because from 1 April – just three months later – matters were being reorganized and the Crewe area would be handed over to another, not least because it was a bit of a trip from my home in Worsley. It was no surprise when, after setting off, I found I couldn't get any further than the entrance to the M6, less than halfway, because of dense fog.

This was back in 1973 when we used to get 'can't-see-the-hand-in-front-of-your-face' fog. The Clean Air Act has seen to it that this is a rarity nowadays but on this occasion driving was impossible. I returned home, telephoned Crewe police station, apologized and explained I would try again in the morning.

Now, potential crime scenes have to remain sterile: you can't have people trampling around all over them. Almost inevitably when the police arc lights go up and the blue lamps on the vehicles are all flashing, a crowd gathers. Given its head that crowd will, understandably, get curious and walk all over the clues. This has to be prevented.

That night, that Christmas Eve, despite the freezing fog that was going to keep all but the most fervent crime-scene junkie indoors, the senior officers knew they had no choice but to make absolutely certain no one interfered with the site. A young bobby was posted at the edge of the wood to repel boarders and spent the night there. He must have loved me.

That Christmas morning was actually rather pleasant, crisp and bright, while still rather cold. It didn't take long to get to Crewe and the police ferried me to the dead man and his circle of bright lights.

He was in a hollow in the wood, just off the road where the bus had passed days earlier, lying face down with the arms underneath the body and the legs partly flexed. He was naked apart from his socks and one shoe. The 'lights' were his other clothes. His left shoe, trousers, shirt, pullover, overcoat, underpants and vest were all strewn about, close to where he lay. At night the dew or the frost would make them shine in the lights of passing cars.

Maggots had got into the body and there was early fungal growth on the skin of the legs and arms. He had clearly been there a few days but to say precisely how long was tricky with the fluctuating daytime and night temperatures that week.

I supervised the removal of the body to Leighton

Hospital and at 11.45 a.m., when most people had completed the opening of their presents and were looking forward to turkey and all the trimmings, I made my first incision.

The corpse was that of Herbert Marshall, fifty-three years of age but looking more like sixty, five feet, four inches tall, with brown hair going grey. The skin was greasy and the side that had been in contact with the ground had an extensive accumulation of soil and leaves. He had a club left foot and the right was missing four toes. Mr Marshall had not found it easy getting around.

The scalp was healthy, the skull intact and while the brain showed putrefaction there was no evidence of any disease or violence.

Marshall had had severe emphysema and the lungs were congested but the pleurae and pleural cavities were healthy. The heart was normal in size and shape but the major arteries and vessels showed moderate arteriosclerosis,

He had nine teeth in his lower jaw and three in the upper, all in a poor state of hygiene. The stomach was empty. There was no sign of violence.

I concluded that he had died of congestive heart failure and that the most likely cause of that was hypothermia. He had been outside in the cold too long and his heart couldn't take it.

This was not a crime so the police were pleased. But it was still a puzzle why Marshall should have removed all his clothes. The toxicology tests and a well-read policeman solved it.

His blood alcohol level was in the region of 200 milligrams, more than three times the driving limit, and would in all probability have been much higher in the time immediately leading up to his death.

Coincidentally, shortly afterwards an officer showed me an article in the *Police Gazette* about a rare condition in which people who are severely under the influence of alcohol can confuse cold with warmth.

We all know how cold can 'burn' but we realize the difference between that kind of burn and the sort from a heat source. Occasionally, the article explained, a befuddled drunk can fail to appreciate the difference and, as he becomes colder, he reacts as if he is getting hotter.

Mr Marshall, we knew, liked his drink and the post-mortem told us he had not been subjected to violence. The eventual conclusion, which the coroner accepted, was that he died from heart failure brought on by alcoholic hypothermia.

Drunk, confused, he had started to get 'warm' as he walked home in the freezing conditions. First off came the overcoat but that brought on more cold – more 'heat' to his addled brain. It would have been as if his clothes were on fire. He ripped them off one by one and cast them aside as he spun around in the clearing before exhaustion and the bitter cold knocked him down and froze him to the bone.

That Christmas the natural cold was as lethal as any cold steel.

14

In Black and White

Fortunately, the random killer is a rarity. The man who will take lives indiscriminately for reasons known only to himself is the most terrifying killer of all because he is beyond any logic, any reason, any civilized argument. One thinks of Michael Ryan at Hungerford using a number of weapons to cut down anyone within range.

But rarely is a crime of extreme violence totally without motive. Ryan may have felt in some twisted manner that the town of Hungerford was his victim. The Yorkshire Ripper's horrors were directed exclusively towards women. And, most dreadful of all, Thomas Hamilton's target at Dunblane – through the destruction of innocent children – was the entire community.

On a much smaller scale, it is often the case that violent people choose to direct their ire at groups or sections within communities instead of at the individuals by whom they feel they have been wronged.

This is an act of cowardice. Instead of dealing with a situation, the attacker cowers from it and, instead, wreaks damage on unsuspecting persons unlikely to give him a hard time. If you confront your enemy you can expect resistance. But if you cheat and attack with no warning a person who has no animosity towards you and no reason to fear that you may strike, the chances are you will win.

These are classic bully tactics.

Identifying a generic group to take the blame for one's failings is often easy. A set of football supporters wearing red, for instance, might not be surprised to fall foul of a group of fans wearing white if the white team has just played the red team and lost to them. This is not to condone such thuggishness. But it is, at least, understandable.

However, if that day fans wearing blue come across the white supporters they might not expect to be attacked. The teams haven't played that day. They have never played. They are in different leagues. But still the whites attack. They attack the colour blue for no better reason than that it is not their own hue.

The peaceful fans have no chance because they are attacked without warning for no good reason and the boot is in before they can defend themselves.

Historically, on the battlefield as now among football yobs, colours were the easiest way of identifying an enemy. Colour, in the singular, is another.

Racist attacks are prevalent in most inner cities. Greater Manchester is said to be the county with the second worst record after Greater London.

Such assaults are based on a nonsense, of course, in that the victim's only crime is that he was born with a different skin shade to the man who is attacking him. The aggressor has decided that the race that this individual represents deserves his retribution. It has absolutely nothing to do with the individual victim. When questioned, the thug can never justify his reasoning other than to spout ill-informed yobbish rhetoric, usually based on jealousy.

The convoluted difficulties arising from racism and criminality have been discussed elsewhere in this book, so we will leave it at that. However, I believe the following two cases go some way towards justifying this simple statement: an act of violence based solely on an individual's racial origin is as abhorrent a crime as it is possible to commit, not least because of its futility and utter stupidity. It is a crime for those at the bottom of the gene pool. The work of morons.

In July 1989 Tahir Akram was fourteen years old and was walking home to Waterloo Street in Oldham hand in hand with his handicapped younger brother when, suddenly, he fell over. A relative saw him collapse, ran to help and found the teenager clutching at his face with his hands, blood oozing between his fingers. He was rushed to hospital but died within half an hour.

When I carried out the post-mortem that same evening it was a puzzle. What had killed him was clear, but how it had happened was less so.

Tahir was a healthy boy in every respect except that a tight group of the arteries and blood vessels at the base of the brain, known as the Circle of Willis, had haemorrhaged and the young man had bled profusely, brain death following on rapidly. Why this should happen was unclear.

There were no marks on the body other than a tiny scrape on his eyelid, close to the eyebrow. It had been noted, but no immediate importance had been attached to it because of its small size. It was the sort of mark you expect to find on lively boys. Initially, the speculation was that he had been struck some kind of blow.

Police inquiries then suggested that there had been a number of shooting incidents in the area around the time Tahir fell. A witness said that the sound of a gunshot, or something like it, had startled him seconds before the youngster collapsed.

There was no immediate evidence that Tahir had been shot but I was able to tell the police that there was documented proof that a sudden, vicious movement of the neck could cause the Willis veins and arteries to rupture. It was rare, but it had been known to happen.

If Tahir had turned suddenly, surprised at such a sound, that could have done it. I have to say, though, that I wasn't really convinced by that theory and neither were the detectives.

We had checked the outside and found no answers. We had examined the inside and found the cause of death but no reason for it. Inside and out. Nowhere else to go – except where it is difficult to get to with a scalpel.

I organized an X-ray, which took a little time. But it proved more than worthwhile and made everything perfectly, horribly, clear. There, in Tahir's head, where it had been for three days, was the airgun pellet. It was the clearest thing on the X-ray slide, a dark, sharp shadow, bullet-shaped behind his eye, nestling in his sinus.

Practically anywhere else and Tahir would have simply run home crying. But the pellet had struck too true. It had entered the eye socket via the tiny hole we had noted earlier and penetrated to a depth of two and a half inches. It had hit no vital organs and hadn't even damaged the eye to which it passed so close. But it had been travelling too fast.

If you throw a stone into a pool of water you see a radiating ripple effect from the point where it lands. It is the same with a bullet. A high-powered rifle can send a projectile clean through a body, missing all vital organs and leaving clean entry and exit wounds on both sides. A similar injury caused by a swordsman's rapier would be no problem. But the shock wave that a speed-of-sound bullet sets in motion causes phenomenal movement within and around the soft tissues to the point where they can begin to break up and cease to function.

In this case, the pellet weight and projectile speed were much lower than those of a rifle bullet. But they struck in a vital area. The shock wave would not have travelled far, but it didn't have to. It was only a matter of a couple of inches to the Circle of Willis, and it shook the vessels till they split.

A crew of dim, drug-using racist yobs from nearby Tameside were arrested and tried for the killing. They had been 'ripped off' by a West Indian for the grand sum of £5 in a cheap drug deal and had decided to avenge themselves on anyone coloured. One black man recalled that shortly before the fatal shot was fired something fired from a car whistled past his ear and the laughing group inside shouted: 'Black bastard'. He was one of three to be fired at before Tahir.

Stephen Lamb, twenty, from Audenshaw, fired all the shots that night. His co-defendants said he told them: 'This will put us on the map.' After spotting the youngster and firing he turned back into the back seat and declared: 'I got one, got one. Blew the back of his head off. Did you see him drop? Like a bag.' The following day he was told the boy had died and responded with astonishing callousness. 'It was only a Paki,' he sneered,

Lamb, a loudmouth, had not blown anyone's head off and probably made the sickening 'Paki' remark out of witless bravado. But his remarks failed to endear him to the jury and his defence that it was all a mistake bore no fruit.

He got life for murder. A twenty-one-year-old accomplice convicted of manslaughter got seven years and two others, aged nineteen and twenty, convicted of lesser charges, were ordered to be detained in a young offenders' institution for three and a half years and six months respectively.

Understandably, the murder raised tensions among the large and sometimes volatile Asian community in Oldham, not least because the police refused to state officially at the time that this was a racially motivated killing. Perhaps the powers-that-be felt that if they denied it then the racial heat would go away. This was a foolish and patronizing attitude that might have resulted in more bloodshed had it not been for one member of the Asian community.

The voice of reason spoke loudly and everyone had to listen. 'I don't feel any hate towards the men who did this, nor any bitterness towards other white people,' the man said. 'We should come closer together and try to understand each other.'

If anyone else had spoken those conciliatory words at that time he might have been shot down in flames for his weakness and foolishness.

In fact, he was showing phenomenal courage, strength, wisdom and community leadership. And no one could deny the right of shopkeeper Mohammed Akram, the father of five children, one of them called Tahir, to speak.

Worthless Wayne Lambert had a pathological hatred of Asians because one of them once got one over on him.

The jobless Londoner had a row with a taxi driver and threatened him but forgot about the cabbie's radio. The intended victim called for help, which soon arrived on the scene. The macho six-footer got some of his own medicine.

A year later Lambert was in Manchester leading a loose group of drug-taking youngsters, including two young girls and a seventeen-year-old boy, in petty crime to feed their amphetamine and heroin habits.

One of the teenagers went into a shop in Withington, Manchester and thought she noticed that the owner, sixty-year-old Mohammed Siddik Dada, had plenty of cash in his pockets.

Minutes later Lambert walked into the shop with the girl and, without saying a word, walked briskly up to the counter. He hit the slightly built shopkeeper hard over the head with an eighteen-inch length of scaffolding pipe he had cut short to fit into his pocket.

The pair searched one pocket but found only £60. They didn't realize the dying man was lying across the other pocket which contained more than £2,000. Most of their loot was spent on health food for fitness freak Lambert. What was left bought a wrap of heroin for the girl.

The following night Lambert and a male cohort were arrested in a stolen Austin Metro and charged with theft. With no evidence to suggest they were anything but car thieves, they were released to take a second life.

The following evening they dialled private hire-taxi firms and ordered cabs. Twice a car arrived but they turned it away, because it had an Afro-Caribbean driver, not an Asian. The third driver to turn up fitted the murderous bill.

It was at two a.m. on Monday, 27 January 1992, that I was invited by police officers to visit Cunard Close, Ardwick, Manchester, where I was shown the body of forty-seven-year-old Mohammed Sarwar Ansari. He was lying face upwards on the road with obvious head injuries and extensive blood staining around the head.

At 4.15 a.m., at Manchester mortuary I measured and weighed him. His face was swollen and distorted, the eyes were swollen and there were lacerations to the chin and from the chin to the lower lip, both one and a half inches long. Further small lacerations in the right eyelid and a larger one to the left side of the forehead were apparent. There was a curved abrasion on the left side of the chest.

The scalp showed extensive bruising and the skull showed severe fractures. There was extensive fracturing of the bones of the face, including nasal bones, both cheek-bones, both upper jaws and the lower jaw in the midline which was broken into several pieces. Several loose teeth were present and the orbits of both eyes were fractured. The surface of the brain showed extensive haemorrhage with petechial haemorrhages in the temporal lobes.

The larynx showed bruising to the right side with a fracture of the right superior horn. Blood was present in the trachea and bronchi, extending into the lungs which also showed inhaled blood.

Mr Ansari had died from severe, heavy blows to the face and head, probably with a blunt instrument. But there was also evidence of either attempted ligature strangulation or blows to the throat and a sustained physical assault on his body.

Mr Dada, in hospital on a life-support machine, was not to succumb to his injuries for more than another week but a murder-level investigation into the assault upon him was well under way. As information poured in, Lambert's name soon featured in both inquiries and he was arrested.

He and his young friends were no match for the interrogators and quickly confessed. Tough guy Lambert cried in his cell. No one cried for him.

Mr Ansari, from Burnage, had picked up the fare and had had no reason to suspect anything when the two men got into the back of his car. He drove them to Cunard Close and as he pulled up Lambert hit him from behind with the scaffolding pole with which he had felled Mr Dada forty-eight hours earlier.

The victim convulsed and was dragged from his vehicle and beaten mercilessly. Lambert then ordered his young accomplice to finish him off and seventeen-year-old petty crook Dean Millington produced a toughened double-pronged toasting fork and jammed it into the defenceless man's face.

As far as hastening their victim's death was concerned, Millington's efforts meant nothing: Mr Ansari's life was already effectively over. His action served merely to increase his own prison sentence. Mr Justice Morland, the judge at Manchester Crown Court, ordered him to be detained during Her Majesty's pleasure for his part in the murder.

Turning to Lambert, he said: 'You were driven by an evil, barbaric, gloating hatred of Pakistanis.' The double killer got life with a recommendation of a twenty-five-year minimum sentence.

After the trial Mr Dada's wife said: 'My only hope after all this is that the public will become aware of some of the terrible racial problems in this country today.

'The loss of my husband was a senseless waste of life. Something must be done to stop or discourage attacks of this kind.'

Is it not remarkable how people in the most tragic circumstances and still stricken by their bereavement can put their pain and anger to one side and speak so eruditely of the greater good? And isn't it a sad and pathetic society that constantly chooses to ignore them?

15

Unsolicited Male

Without wanting to appear too blasé, I have to admit that not too much surprises me these days. Very early in my career I came to the conclusion that people are capable of committing phenomenally strange and imaginative acts of violence upon each other.

However, I was taken aback somewhat when awakened quite early on a Sunday morning by the ringing of the bedside telephone and a policeman with a heavy Lancashire accent growling the immortal words: 'Ay, Doc, someone's shoved a penis through a letter box.'

A mother and her daughter had got the attention of the desk sergeant when they had walked into his police station in Bolton and presented him with the offending object.

The women had found the bloodied article on the mat when they had come down for breakfast. They had taken it immediately to the station in a state of some distress and considerable fury.

Understandably, the two women were beside themselves with outrage. The idea that someone could leave a penis on their hall floor was an absolute disgrace and they made it perfectly clear they wanted something done about it.

But perhaps because of the shocking nature of their morning surprise, they did not appear to have made a connection between the severed organ and its former owner. Rather, they seemed to see the penis as an entity in itself.

The policeman, with his years of training, was fully aware that people rarely become detached from their genitalia on purpose. Out there was someone who was either severely injured or dead, probably the latter. Hence the call to me.

By the time I reached the police station on 16 April 1972, they had found the rest of him – or, to be more accurate, most of the rest of him.

Detectives took me to a demolition area in Lorne Street, Farnworth, where rows of terraced houses were being destroyed and rubble was piled everywhere. I was directed to a derelict outside toilet.

At the entrance an adult male, fully clothed, was lying on his back with his face upwards. There were extensive bloodstains around the head, his trousers were torn and the front of his abdomen was exposed, revealing a number of transverse incisions – and an amputation of the penis.

Blood was present on the wall of the outhouse and on the ground outside and there were marks in the ground suggesting the victim had been dragged. When the body was removed bloodstains and pieces of brain became apparent where the head had been lying.

At the mortuary at the Bolton and District General Hospital the post-mortem on James Alexander Scott, aged sixty-four, began, as usual, with an external examination. He was unusually small in stature, just five feet tall.

There were lacerations, bruises and abrasions to both sides of his face, his nose and the back of his head. On the front of the neck were two lacerations, one of which cut right through the skin, but there was no reaction or bleeding from this pair of wounds.

The front of the abdomen showed seven transverse cuts over an area three and a half inches deep around the umbilicus, one of which penetrated through to the abdominal cavity. These were also bloodless and, like the previously mentioned pair, appeared to have been caused after death. A further, larger laceration in the perineum, also post-mortem, had removed the penis. The right testicle was present but the left was missing. It was never found.

There was a further one-inch laceration on the left thigh across the groin and numerous small abrasions on the front of both legs and the backs of the hands. There were bruises on the knuckle of the left thumb and below the right thumb. Further scrape marks and abrasions were found on the back.

Nothing to do with his death, of course, but it was obvious that Mr Scott had also suffered quite badly from piles.

I was given the penis that had been handed in at the police station. It matched against the laceration on the body, apart from the lack of a left testicle.

Internally, the skull showed evidence of a ferocious attack. There were extensive fractures to the frontal and parietal bones which were more pronounced on the left side than the right. The front of the skull was shattered, with the destruction of both eye orbits and the upper jaw on each side. The base of the skull was fractured and the pituitary fossa destroyed. The nasal bones were fractured, the meninges were torn on the left side and there was laceration of the brain substance on the left side. The brain showed surface haemorrhage, laceration of the left cerebral hemisphere and petechial haemorrhages in both cerebral hemispheres.

The bones of the larynx were fractured on both sides and the trachea and bronchi contained inhaled blood. There were petechial haemorrhages in the eyes.

Police asked me for my version of the chain of events in this attack as indicated by the findings of the post-mortem examination.

I decided the assault probably began a little distance away from the outhouse, with the victim being grasped around the neck in a stranglehold with pressure sufficiently firm to fracture the bones of the larynx. The eye haemorrhages suggested strangulation had taken place but I considered this pressure would not have been maintained for more than thirty seconds. If it had been continued for any longer than that length of time it would probably have resulted in death, but clearly some of the other injuries had been sustained while the victim was still alive.

The pressure would have lasted long enough for Mr Scott to slip into unconsciousness and to cause the sphincters of his body to relax, indicated by the soiling of his trousers with the contents of the bowel.

Scrape marks on the ground at the outhouse suggested that the helpless man was then dragged across the site close to the building to a point where significant bloodstaining was later found. Here was where he received at least eight hard blows to the head that were of such intensity they shattered the bones that make up the face and skull. Death would have occurred rapidly from the damage to the brain and from haemorrhage.

Detectives were later to establish that the murder weapon was a brick, or a number of bricks.

The bruising on the face – a reaction to the punishment his body was receiving – showed that he was not dead when the blows began to rain down on him. However, he was certainly dead by the time that stage of the assault was concluded. Add to this the eye haemorrhages, which are a reaction to strangulation, and these two facts together told me that the strangulation must have occurred first. But it failed to kill him and was followed by the battery of the head, which was terminal.

The dead body was then thrown into the outhouse, the force of its landing resulting in the brains and blood being spilled out onto the floor to be found only when we moved the head.

After death the body was subjected to mutilation with a knife, with ten superficial cuts and the amputation of the penis. The lack of reaction to these wounds proves they had to be post-mortem.

As in so many cases of murder, Mr Scott, a shy, lonely bachelor who would not, indeed could not, hurt anyone had died because he was in the wrong place at the wrong time and had met someone who was drunk, angry and with a natural inclination towards cowardly violence.

Melvyn Harrison, aged twenty-two, who lived in Lorne Street, had taken a bus that evening to visit the Nightingale Inn in Bolton where he and a friend met up with two girls whom they knew. After a lot of beer they missed their last bus and all of them had to walk home to Farnworth.

Harrison kissed one of the girls goodnight and asked her for a date. No doubt unimpressed with his technique she refused point-blank and he went away seething.

Around the corner, Mr Scott had enjoyed a few drinks himself at his local, The Railway, and walked down Egerton Street to a fish-and-chip shop where he bought a chicken breast to take home for his dog.

On his way he had the misfortune to bump into Harrison who knew the old man and had noticed he occasionally splashed out generously with his money in The Railway. He decided to rob him and, as they walked past the demolition area, the younger man struck without warning.

Harrison was in his own house within seconds of the murder. But it was two hours later that he hatched his sickening and perverse plan to wreak vengeance on the young woman who had spurned his advances.

He returned to the body with a knife, tore the trousers and chopped away until he had removed the penis. He then carried it a few hundred yards to the girl's house and posted it gleefully through the letter box.

This act, while providing Harrison with warped satisfaction, also sealed his fate.

As soon as the girl told the police about her walk home with Harrison the night before and her refusal of his advances they had their chief suspect. He rapidly confessed.

At Liverpool Crown Court Harrison admitted manslaughter but denied murder on the grounds that he did not intend to do his victim serious harm. My opinion about the ferocity of the attack helped the jury find him guilty of murder and the judge sentenced him to life.

Forensic evidence about the brick used to batter the victim was provided by Dr Alan Clift, an expert later discredited over other cases.

At a subsequent appeal Harrison's lawyers tried to suggest Dr Clift's evidence was unsafe or unsatisfactory. However, Lord Lane, the Lord Chief Justice, sitting with two other judges, declared that, because of the weight of pathological evidence provided by me at the trial, it would not have made a 'ha' p'orth of difference' to the outcome if Dr Clift had never been called as a witness at all.

While the nature of the previous crime made it among the most strange I have encountered, it was the *place* of the next that was unusual.

Prestbury is probably still considered to be the most salubrious place to live in the North-West of England. Never flash but always quietly superior with an old-world veneer, it traded for decades on the fact that it was mentioned in the Domesday Book. In the 1970s this large village was a place where both genuinely 'old' money and – much to that group's dismay – the nouveaux riches of advertising, PR and TV collaborated to send the prices of houses into orbit.

More recently it has become the retreat of some of the more famous Premier League footballers. Whether this fact in time returns the prices of the real estate to more sensible levels remains to be seen.

But in 1977 this was a very smart, very law-abiding and very peaceful place. Although firmly in the North-West where the vowels were exceedingly long and the pedigrees of the residents even longer, it was as safe as the safest Home Counties suburbs.

On a cold Friday afternoon in February a lady in her late middle age parked her car in the picturesque main road, walked a few yards along the High Street to the white-painted office of Williams and Glyn's Bank and was disappointed to discover that it was closed. Mildly irritated, she breathed a heavy sigh, returned to her car, set it in gear and drove to another branch in nearby Macclesfield. In Prestbury mild irritation was as furious as one was expected to get: one didn't get annoyed, that would have been unseemly.

At Macclesfield, completely calm, she picked up her cash and, on departing, casually mentioned to the cashier that she thought the Prestbury branch was normally open on a Friday afternoon. The teller, aware that the lady customer was from Prestbury, knew full well that the branch she referred to was certainly open on Friday afternoons. Clearly the lady was confused, had gone to the wrong door, and had lacked the strength to open it. Or maybe she had made the whole thing up. But he merely smiled politely and said he'd check on it.

He told his boss who telephoned the office and, perplexingly, got no reply. The Post Office confirmed the line was in order. Now worried, they then contacted estate agents J. R. Bridgford who had the shop next door to the Prestbury office and whose staff they knew well and asked them to check it out. The estate agents found what the lady had discovered. The place was locked.

By now it was fifty-six minutes after the branch should have reopened following the staff's lunch break. Two clerks from Macclesfield were dispatched with spare keys. Fifteen minutes later they were on the telephone in hysterics.

The office had two staff, senior clerk Ian Jebb, twenty-two, who was engaged to be married, and his assistant Susan Hockenhull, nineteen years old and said to be somewhat shy and timid.

They found Ian. He was dead on the floor of the office. They didn't find Susan. She had vanished, along with about £2,500.

At no point did anyone believe that Susan was responsible either for Ian's death or the missing money. This was a case of murder and kidnapping.

I arrived at 5.20 p.m. and was shown Ian's body lying face up behind the bank counter in pools of blood, with splashes under the counter and on the wall behind his head. A cloth gag was across his mouth and his hands had been tied behind his back.

The body was removed to the West Park Hospital, Macclesfield. It was 6.30 p.m. and rigor mortis was already starting to develop in the limbs. The body temperature was thirty degrees Centigrade. This would help to establish the time of death, which had occurred not long previously.

Ian Jebb was not a big man, five feet, three inches tall, and clothed in a waistcoat, shirt, underpants, trousers, socks and shoes. The gag was secured by a single knot below the left ear. The hands had been tied with twin-flex electric cable.

The waistcoat showed two cuts on the front left side, another at the front right side, two at the back and one on the left shoulder.

There was a superficial cut a little over an inch long in the left upper eyelid and a significant wound, one and a half inches deep, below the right ear. The back of the head showed three ragged lacerations on the left side of the occipital area, each around an inch in length.

The front of the chest showed two lacerations, both of which had penetrated for at least two and a half inches.

On the back were a further two wounds and all four appeared to have been caused by a double-edged knife.

The hands and wrists showed constriction marks corresponding to the flex that had been tied around the hands.

Internally, the scalp had bruising in the left occipital area and the brain was oedematous. Ian had been hit over the head twice, possibly three times. This did not kill him.

The chest had a wound three inches long between the fourth and fifth ribs caused by a combination of two of the wounds mentioned earlier. This entered the pericardium and the front of the heart causing a transverse wound two and a half inches long. It entered both the right and left ventricles, cut the interventricular septum and damaged the mitral valve. This would have been swiftly fatal.

There were two puncture wounds to the left side close to the vertebral bodies between the fifth and sixth ribs and the seventh and eighth ribs, both of which entered the lower lobe of the lungs.

It was clear that Ian had died around one o'clock on the afternoon of 25 February, only five and a half hours before I began my post-mortem examination. He had been hit over the head with a blunt instrument, tied and gagged, and then stabbed at the front and back of the chest, probably while in a sitting position, helpless and utterly terrified. The stabs were directed downwards and inwards with considerable force, using a double-edged knife with a blade at least three inches long and a little over one inch wide We were to discover that, even in these appalling circumstances, Ian Jebb was that day much luckier than his friend.

At the moment I was deciding her colleague's cause of death Susan Hockenhull was shivering alone in the cold, high on a moor with darkness closing in. The undiluted horror that this young, tender girl had experienced as she witnessed what had happened in the bank would have changed to overwhelming terror at what was now happening to her. She would have been unable to move, was probably in pain and living through a genuinely diabolical nightmare that was to end with her death.

Both Susan and Ian knew the man who killed them and probably regarded him as nearly a friend, certainly an acquaintance with whom they would have been happy to share the time of day and a cup of tea. Outwardly, like most human monsters, David Walsh appeared perfectly normal.

He was one of triplets who, within three months of their birth in 1946 in Chesterfield, Derbyshire, were abandoned by their parents and sent to orphanages. In 1961 he began work as a car-wash attendant and a year later tried his hand as an apprentice welder. But that didn't work out. He was subsequently sacked by the Coal Board for continuously taking time off and failed to hold down a job in a machine shop for the same reason. At age seventeen he joined the Army but the Royal Engineers decided after a year that he was 'undesirable'. In between long bouts of unemployment or imprisonment for petty theft he took a variety of uninteresting jobs, none of which lasted. Some he held down for no longer than a single day.

In 1972 he found something that interested him, repairing business adding machines, and during the following four years he worked for six different companies, travelling around. Not only did he enjoy the work, it allowed him to indulge his passion for fast driving, which, inevitably, also got him into trouble with the law. During a fourteen-month period before the murders while he lived in Macclesfield with his wife Linda, he was seen driving a Ford Escort van, a mini-van, a 750cc motorbike, an Austin 1100 and an Austin Maxi. Yet he was in debt.

Only a few days before the killings he had been handed an eviction notice by bailiffs because of rent arrears of £37.25. He also owed £464 for a Honda bike, £729 for a Rover car and £40 on a loan. At that time, for Walsh, this added up to big money.

A friend recalled how Walsh had bragged that if he was to rob a bank it would be the Williams and Glyn's in Prestbury because it had lousy security. He knew the premises because he regularly serviced its machines. And, of course, he knew the people who worked there. The trouble was: they knew him, too.

Less than four hours after the bank staff found Ian dead and Susan missing, Walsh paid off his £40 debt in cash. Later that evening he bought Linda a Mini for £380 in £10 notes. The following day he went on a spending spree, buying a cassette radio, a guitar and a pair of earrings. Walsh was suddenly flush. He had been given £800 by a pal, he explained.

While he was spending his crisp bank-fresh notes, Susan's frantic family were waiting for news of their daughter. A massive police hunt to find her was under way and everyone knew that, if she was out of doors, they were racing against time. A phone call was made to police, probably by Walsh in a momentary recurrence of conscience, and the anonymous voice told them where she could be found. It was twenty-four hours since she had vanished and, in the circumstances, during that bitterly cold February with ground temperatures falling as low as minus seven degrees Centigrade, twenty-four hours was far too long.

Susan had been walked from the bank to Walsh's Maxi saloon and driven fifteen miles almost due south along the main A523 route, through Macclesfield, into Staffordshire and up onto the bleak upland moors above the town of Leek. Walsh made a left turn and climbed up a minor road towards Meerbrook, 1,200 feet above sea level and well above the snowline. Finally he parked the car and walked her along a farm track, popular in summer as a lovers' lane but normally deserted in winter. They crossed two fields and stopped by a wall. Scars later found on Susan's knees and knuckles suggested that she had been dragged along the ground, so she may have been already bound in some way at this stage.

When Susan was found she was tied in a complex ligature that secured her hands behind her back but was also connected to a fastening around her neck, the whole design producing a tension in the bonds. While there was no evidence of strangulation, the binding would have made it impossible for her to move her arms or head significantly as any movement would have tightened the hold on her throat, thus causing breathing problems. Her ankles were also tied to ensure she couldn't walk. She couldn't have moved at all. She was gagged and so could not call out for help, but then there was no one to hear her. All she could do was wait, immobile, staring at the moor and the gathering night.

Susan had left the bank without her coat and shoes so she was clad only in her indoor working clothes and was barefoot. The biting cold would have been very unpleasant at the time she was abandoned, mid-afternoon. Snow was still falling in occasional light flurries. At one stage while he was with her Walsh removed his own jacket and pullover. Susan might have thought he was going to give them to her so she could stay warm, but he did not. Instead he tore them up and used the strips to bind her. The clothing would later be damning evidence against him.

My colleague Dr Alan Usher handled the post-mortem as Susan's body was discovered within his jurisdiction. He found no signs of violence other than the marks on her knees and knuckles and no sign of sexual interference. He concluded that she froze to death.

Typically in such cases one would expect to notice pink patches on the skin, characteristically distributed around large joints and on the face. Also there might be swelling around the ankles.

Internally there is oedema of the lungs and the lining of the stomach may show shallow acute ulcers. Also, over the pancreas, patches of yellow fat necrosis may be seen extending onto the adjacent mesentery.

In the event neither his findings nor mine were challenged by the defence. Ian died from stab wounds and Susan died from hypothermia.

Clearly Susan could have identified Walsh and had witnessed him commit murder, so when the pair left the bank he knew she was a massive threat to his freedom. His choice was simple: he could let her go, in which case he would go to jail, or he could kill her, in which case she would not be able to provide evidence against him. It is clear that he decided upon the second course but it must be said that it would have been much kinder if he had had the cold courage to give her the swift death he had given her colleague at the bank.

While an initial check of the crime scene was made as soon as Ian's body was discovered, the search for Susan, still possibly alive, was so frantic that detailed examination of the bank premises was put back until the following day. (Nowadays crime scenes are always sealed, sometimes for a full twenty-four hours, to preserve clues and ensure potential evidence is not compromised.)

In the initial search police noticed that sandwiches, an iced bun and a packet of crisps, clearly lunch brought by either of the two victims or the killer, were on a desk, half eaten. Bite marks in the bread could be a vital clue. Little else of obvious significance was spotted.

But when detectives went in the morning after to carry out their meticulous search of the premises they discovered two remarkable things. The sandwiches had inexplicably disappeared but, startlingly, a constable found ransom notes that had been screwed up and thrown in the waste bin. One of them read: '£20,000 and the girl goes free.'

Chief Superintendent Gerald Williams, the senior officer handling the inquiry, rightly went ballistic and demanded to know how one piece of potential evidence could vanish from a murder scene and how another piece, massively important, could be missed in the first checks.

The answer lay in the bored mind of a young police officer. PC Justin Hardy, aged twenty, the son of a judge with promotion on his mind, had been tasked with protecting the scene and left alone in the premises all night. To pass the time he played mind games and put himself in the killer's shoes, trying to imagine what was going on in the man's mind. He scribbled ransom notes in a manner he considered the desperate murderer-thief might have considered and tossed them in the wastepaper basket. Then, hungry, he took a long look at the sandwiches – and ate the evidence. Wisely, he resigned from the Cheshire Constabulary.

The food was not necessary to convict Walsh, nor would the ransom notes have been required even if they'd been genuine. The other evidence against him was massive and he got life, with a recommendation that he serve at least twenty-five years. Sometimes a quarter of a century can seem such a short length of time.

16

Heat

Until the Manchester Airport disaster, the tragedy at the Summerland entertainment complex on the Isle of Man was the most cataclysmic fire on British soil since World War Two.

Fifty people died and, as with all such disasters, it happened because of a series of mistakes and a set of unfortunate circumstances. It is understandable, even correct, that angry and bereaved people should look for someone to blame when there is such an appalling loss of life, but rarely is it the fault of any one individual, never is there one single, overriding cause. You might as well scream at the wind about this tragedy, for here, as on the tarmac at Manchester, one of the culprits was the weather.

It was the late 1960s and in the North-West of England it was raining. Entrepreneurial travel companies were selling packages to take families abroad to guaranteed sunshine and the Brits came running. It was just as easy to get everyone to the airport and then let the reps take the strain as it was to get the train to Morecambe or Blackpool – or to take the ferry over to the Isle of Man and stay at a boarding house. It wasn't even much more expensive when you consider the price of Spanish or Greek beer. Foreigners had not yet got round to ripping off tourists. And 'abroad' was sunny and glamorous.

Back home the beleaguered tourist boards and town councils that relied on summer visitors realized they had to do something about this new trend. The idea of Summerland – a giant fun palace for families – was embraced enthusiastically by everyone who was anyone in the island's capital, Douglas.

It cost two million pounds to build, and was the biggest building on the Isle of Man and the largest entertainment structure in Europe. Against the odds, they managed to get it completed and open just in time for the summer season of 1971. It was an instant success and grew in popularity until the night of 2 August 1973, when there were 3,000 staff, locals and holiday-makers in the place.

The building had a basement for storage and maintenance above which a huge ground floor was laid out like a massive promenade, complete with deck chairs. Upstairs were three vast balconies: on the first level was the marquee show bar, from which stairs led up again to the leisure terrace and further still to what was called the 'cruise deck'.

The use of terracing rather than conventional floors gave an awesome feeling of space, with the roof way up in the sky. There were bars, restaurants, amusement machines and several areas for children to play. Safely, they said.

And it was sunny. The clever design had the walls panelled with a transparent plastic sheeting called Oroglass. At first – not least because I found large quantities of the stuff clogging the throats of the dead – this substance was blamed for the disaster since people assumed it was the burning plastic that caused the fire to blaze with such devastating power. In fact, while the

Oroglass sheets were far from ideal for such a building and should never have been used, they did not ignite until sixteen minutes after the fire began and then only at a very high temperature.

The problem was not only with the Oroglass but also with several other features of the design and the inappropriate materials that were used.

The fire began outside the main building when three youths set fire – they said with a cigarette end – to a plastic hut on the minigolf course. It collapsed against Summerland's south-east wall, which was made of a form of corrugated metal sheeting called Galbestos. On the original plans this wall was to have been built from reinforced concrete but that would have been more expensive and costs – as with any major building project – were a factor no one could ignore.

Inside the building a hessian-covered screen made out of inflammable fibreboard was erected close to the Galbestos exterior wall. This created a gap fourteen inches wide and sixteen feet high that acted like a chimney, drawing in the fire from outside. It continued to burn and grow in power behind the screen, hidden from the unsuspecting throng within.

Some smoke filtered into the main area but no one reacted. It transpired that practically none of the staff had been trained in fire drill. A full sixteen minutes after the blaze had begun it burst through into the ground-floor amusement arcade and within less than three more minutes the arcade was an inferno. Several people did try to start the fire-alarm system but for some reason it failed to work.

The fire spread like an inverted rolling waterfall,

travelling upwards instead of down. When the arcade downstairs became engulfed and the flames hit the rear wall they kicked back, hungrily seeking out more oxygen.

Working their way from the back of the room, fiery fingers picked their way erratically forwards along the ceiling like fast red and yellow spiders. When they reached the end of the terrace they gripped the edge ferociously, curled upwards and around in an acrobatic arc, landed on the front of the next floor and began to consume what was before them.

And when that tier was done two others beckoned.

Insatiable, the fire took everything in its path. First the ground floor, then the marquee show bar, after that the leisure terrace and finally the cruise deck were all absorbed by its fearsome power.

Inside the wall cavity the fire continued to spread horizontally and found a second 'chimney' space twenty-four inches wide between the end of the terraces and the Oroglass wall. The 'chimney' stretched from the floor to the roof and the flames shot up it, igniting the plastic sheets of the upper walls and ceiling and turning them into fireballs from the sky.

Interestingly, By-law 39 on the Isle of Man insists that external walls should be made of material that will resist fire for at least two hours. But in 1967 the Douglas Corporation and the Isle of Man Local Government Board agreed that it should be waived as far as the Summerland Development was concerned.

Further regulations that laid down rules for places of entertainment about fire doors, fire escapes and so on were also ignored. Summerland was the answer to the local holiday industry's prayers and a few regulations created by petty bureaucrats were not going to prevent its development.

Another mistake was to forget to take into account a psychological factor affecting people's attempts to escape from the fire. This was a place where parents and kids went their separate ways for entertainment. It was designed 'for all'. When the blaze ripped through the wall the parents didn't make for the fire exits, they made for their children. This meant that during the panic people were trying to go in opposite directions on the same stair-cases. Several fell and the speed of escape for all was drastically reduced.

From the second terrace there was a concrete-protected fire escape but most people ran towards the open stair-cases with which they were familiar. Even six of those who chose correctly to make for the fire escape perished through awful luck. The fire never reached them but they were asphyxiated when a member of staff turned the power off, the lights went out and they stumbled in the darkness. The lights should have had a back-up system. It failed.

The staircases were made of wood and when they collapsed there were still more than twenty people on them, trying to make their way to safety. Too late.

Of the fifty dead, nine were children.

It was necessary to identify each of the victims through the examination of dental records. This job was carried out by Dr J. Ken Holt from the dental hospital and since, unlike at the Manchester disaster, there was no passenger list from which to establish the identities of those killed, formal identification was a very long and complex task.

I arrived the evening after the fire and went straight to

the hospital to meet up with the local pathologist, Dr Stephen Baker. We were later joined by another mainland colleague, Dr John Benstead, and a team of forensic scientists including the unfortunate Frank Skuse, later to be castigated over his involvement in the prosecution of the Birmingham Six.

The following morning I visited the site while they were still retrieving bodies. There were many people milling about, some working in the wreckage and others just standing, watching in shocked bewilderment. As at Ringway there was a heavy, almost palpable silence and a feeling of absolute desolation.

I noticed many curtains were still in place, but now they were open to the elements and fluttering in the breeze. Whilst the fire had done wholesale damage the swimming pool was still intact, though now with splodges of gum scattered over its water's surface like so many dead fish.

This fire, like all large fires, had moved around inside the building almost like a being with a personality, taking some things whole but just scratching peevishly at others. Quite a lot of the wooden beams used on the staircases, while blackened on the surface, were hardly affected underneath. In the pocket of one dead little boy we found an undamaged bar of chocolate.

We worked in a line on three tables and shared out the work fairly evenly. The pathology was essentially uneventful and in each case the cause of death was inhalation of fumes. We got blood from every body and the level of carbon monoxide was almost identical throughout, around seventy-five to eighty per cent. This is a fatal level.

The only unusual thing was that in the throats of all the dead was a revolting sticky goo, the remains of the Oroglass. It had separated in the intense heat and become tiny particles of floating plastic that filled the atmosphere and was inhaled by those who failed to get out in time. Once it had been hard plastic forming the sides of a giant building but when I found it, one and a half days later, it was still messy and soft. It didn't actually kill anyone but it would have been a dreadful experience as it clogged the throats of the fifty already suffering from the effects of carbon monoxide poisoning.

It was the first disaster of this magnitude in the country for a very long time so the sheer logistics of dealing with so many bodies posed practical problems. Noble's Hospital on the island was in the process of building a new mortuary and there was insufficient storage space for the dead. Eventually it was decided to use a nearby school.

Each corpse was brought into the mortuary, examined and then taken by ambulance from our rooms to the school. Someone had the bright idea of using sleeves of plastic to wrap the bodies. They arrived as large tubes, open at each end like a sausage case. The bodies were placed inside in formaldehyde to preserve them and then both ends were sealed.

Mr Justice Cantley chaired a three-month public inquiry that pinpointed many of the mistakes and errors of judgement that had exacerbated the situation but concluded: 'There were no "villains".'

At the inquest, the coroner, Henry Callow, instructed the jury: 'The evidence disclosed in this inquiry would not justify a finding of criminal negligence.' So directed, the jury of seven men returned a verdict of death by misadventure on all fifty victims.

A spokesman for the families voiced disagreement with the authorities' opinions. 'There *were* villains,' he said. 'This was an unparalleled disaster caused by local government negligence, lack of concern and a complete disregard of building regulations and fire-safety precautions on the part of highly paid experts and senior executives.'

Whatever the truth, whether or not any one person or small group was criminally responsible for this disaster, the record shows that there were three prosecutions arising from it. Three schoolboys from Liverpool, one aged fourteen and two aged twelve, pleaded guilty to causing wilful damage to a plastic kiosk on the miniature golf course at Summerland.

Each was fined three pounds.

At lunchtime on 8 May 1979, in the Woolworth's store in Piccadilly Gardens, Manchester, around seventy people were sitting down to their meals in the restaurant on the second floor.

Many of the diners were regulars who used the place to meet up for a chat. They'd put their shopping down under the tables and lean across, swapping gossip and small talk. They were mostly women but there were also families and, occasionally, a pair of men. This was the restaurant's busiest time.

The large room was open-plan and a five-feet-tall partition separated the eating area from the rest of the floor, much of which was devoted to selling furniture, mostly suites. Several of these were piled high at the back of the room, against a wall, ready to be bought and transported.

Various displays were illuminated to show them off to their best advantage, the intention to catch the eye of any potential buyer. The lamps were powered through a system of extension wires leading back to several plugs that had been connected to a single electric socket on the far side of the room. The socket itself was hidden from view behind the stacks of chairs and sofas.

While that was where the fire started, it is not known whether that heavily loaded socket and its spaghetti junction of wiring was the cause. A frayed wire or discarded cigarette could also have been responsible – we never found out. But, however the fire began, the view of those seated behind the partition was too obscured for them to notice its first sudden flare.

When the flames were spotted by staff a number acted promptly, both to tackle the blaze with extinguishers and to warn the customers. But no one rang the Fire Brigade. The nearest fire station was 300 yards away in London Road but as the fire spread with surprising speed and the amateurs were forced back the professionals had no reason to stir. Their first call was from a passing taxi driver who noticed smoke and used his radio to get his control to dial 999.

As is so often the case in the early stages of desperate situations, many people failed to recognize the seriousness and immediacy of the danger. A cashier started to cash up rather than run but was quickly ordered by her boss to forget about the money and get out. She did as she was told and headed for the exit. She lived.

Advised by an agitated assistant to leave everything and move, a seventy-year-old man looked up from his meal, irritably informed her that he had only just ordered his soup and turned back to his food. Within a minute a dark blanket of smoke descended like a theatre safety curtain and separated him from the fleeing throng. He died.

He was one of ten who lost their lives that afternoon in a fire that was to have far-reaching implications for the design of department stores, as well as serious effects on the furniture trade.

New laws were brought in to curb the deadly poisonous effects of highly inflammable polyurethane foam used as filling in the production of modern furniture. Scandalously, a full fifteen years after these terrible deaths, those laws were shown to have been flouted regularly through the use of unchecked, cheap foreign imports. I fervently hope that the current situation is significantly better in all our shops, offices and homes. One would have thought that the difference between life and death was sufficient incentive.

'Woolies' was a national institution – even though it was originally an American firm. It felt comfortable, trustworthy, and many folk swore by it. It was a friendly place, a shop designed for the no-nonsense class. You got bargains and you didn't get ripped off at Woolies. In every sense the shopper was safe there.

In the previous few months there had been a number of improvements, refurbishments and extensions to the store, which was very much a landmark in Manchester. These should have resulted in more stringent fire precautions but, while the company had not yet got a valid fire certificate, the Brigade had been round to check if everything was up to scratch.

They prepared a list of things that needed to be addressed but the law allowed a generous period of time for the safety systems to be put in place. Woolworth's also successfully applied for a number of extensions to the deadlines. It was normal practice then. It may still be, I don't know.

There was no sprinkler system. A later inquiry was to suggest that overhead water sprayers would have saved some if not all of the casualties from their fate. But, while the company prided itself on always adhering to local authority guidelines and some of its other stores had sprinklers, in the case of Manchester there was no such requirement.

The fire rapidly took hold in the area of the stacked furniture. The wooden frames hardly had time to ignite before the polyurethane filling and polypropylene used in the manufacture of the covers were belching out thick, black smoke, crammed with carbon monoxide, carbon dioxide and cyanide. While the CO_2 was non-poisonous it had the effect of smothering any pockets of oxygen that those choking for breath might have located. The other two gases were killers in their own right.

In a scientific test it was shown that when flames were applied to similar furniture it took less than thirty seconds for the room temperature to increase from a perfectly pleasant sixty-six degrees Fahrenheit to a non-survivable 1,500 degrees. A second test raised the temperature to an even greater 1,900°F. In both tests flames reached more than forty feet in height.

Further re-creations of the situation showed that sufficient smoke was released to contaminate the whole of the upper half of the Woolworth store's second floor within just sixty seconds and to fill the entire volume of that part of the store within two minutes.

Most people tend to react at about the same speed. As

shoppers began to grasp the significance of what was happening, they moved together towards the exits, inadvertently causing logjams as they tried to squeeze out of the doorways.

One elderly woman tried to drag her brother to safety but he had a serious heart condition and didn't have the strength or the speed to cope with the jostling crowd. He got caught in the mill of people behind and she had to let go of his hand. As she stumbled out into the light and the safety of the street she expected him to be a few heads behind her but when she turned to look for him he wasn't there.

The brave lady had to be physically prevented from going back to look for him. Those who restrained her did the right thing for by this time her brother, whose body was found later, slumped on the second floor, would have been dead.

The only member of staff to die was a sixty-eight-year-old cleaner who was last seen at the top of an escalator ushering customers down to safety in front of him. His body, covered in debris, was the last to be found by firemen.

Apart from his, all the other bodies were located in a small area between the restaurant and a fire door leading to stairs. The three youngest victims, two women and a man aged twenty-eight, twenty-nine and thirty-one, piled on top of each other, were just six feet from what would have been survival.

Each of the ten victims died from the effects of inhaling fumes rather than from the fire itself. Toxicology tests showed a mixture of high levels of carbon monoxide and cyanide in their blood. It would have been a matter of seconds between inhalation and unconsciousness. Those who died were on the second floor but several people were rescued from upper floors and the roof after running there to escape. The Fire Brigade was there in time for them. As well as the fatalities a further forty-eight people were injured.

The furniture that burned and gave off the killing gases complied with the British Standard at the time even though everyone knew it was highly inflammable and was claiming 100 lives a year in house fires.

It took a further nine years – and several more furniture-related deaths – before legislation was passed that brought in new rules about production and labelling.

In 1994 a survey by Trading Standards Officers found that a third of upholstered furniture examined in 118 shops throughout Greater Manchester broke these laws.

Two years earlier seven mothers aged between twenty-four and thirty-eight arrived for work at an office block in China Lane, just around the corner from Woolworth's, at six p.m. The unusual start time suited them as they could go out when their husbands got home from their jobs and the men could take over looking after the children. Between them the women had eighteen children.

They worked for a company that produced punch cards for computers, Northern Punch Bureau, and theirs was known as the 'married women's shift'.

As they each walked through the ground-floor entrance to the building, Murray House, none could have known that a fire was already burning in a chip shop in the basement. It had started, for a reason never determined, under a worktop in the sandwich-bar section. The fire grew steadily in intensity but was held back by a partition wall in the basement and then by the asbestos lining on the stairwell and fire doors.

It did not burst through until all the women were fifty feet higher up on the top floor, their punch-card machines loud enough to drown out the crackling sound of approaching flames.

The workers knew there was a fire escape just five paces from the door of their office which would certainly have helped them to escape. But they never reached it.

We will never know why for sure, but one possibility is that the smoke, which was ahead of the fire on this high level, billowed up the stairs or along whichever space it could find and, on reaching the fifth floor, surged down the corridor so quickly that it blocked off their route. They were the only people in the entire building: everyone else in the other nine firms on various floors had gone home, so there was no one below to raise the alarm before the smoke got so frighteningly close.

Even as the fumes came at them they could still have escaped unaided if they had held their breath, walked blind into the smoke, felt their way to the door and got out. But that, of course, is much easier said than done. Instead, they retreated across their small room to the point furthest away from the smoke, away from the door, away from the corridor – and away from the fire escape. They backed up to a window, opened it and, while six screamed for help, the seventh dialled 999.

At 6.48 p.m. the emergency switchboard operator at the Dial House exchange received the call and put it through to the control room of the London Road fire station, itself almost within shouting distance of Murray House.

The woman's voice on the line was hysterical and there was a great deal of background noise and shouting that made it impossible for either the Post Office operator or the listening fire officer to get a fix on the address of the emergency.

They managed to make out the words 'fire' and 'lane'. But the interference noise got steadily louder and the caller's voice more high-pitched until she screamed and the line went dead. The conversation, which, like all emergency calls, was recorded on tape, had lasted precisely twenty-nine seconds.

At 6.51 p.m. a second call was received from someone outside the building who had noticed smoke pouring from a window. The yells of the women could be heard clearly by people in the street and several passers-by caught glimpses of them as they waved their arms in desperation.

But the inferno was now raging on the first and second floors, producing flames and choking fumes that were surging out of the shattered windows, sending black clouds climbing up the side of the building, hiding the married women's shift from view.

It took just sixty seconds for the first firemen to get to the scene but by then there were flames visible on all five floors – and the screaming had stopped. They tried to use a forty-five-foot ladder to climb up to where they had been told people were trapped but flames issuing from the lower-floor windows made that impossible.

The fire was too intense for men to get up through the inside of the building so three officers wearing breathing apparatus climbed up the fire escape on the outside of the office block while a turntable ladder was rigged to reach the top storey.

The men on the ladder made it just ahead of the climbers. They found three prone figures to the left of the window and three to the right. The last woman lay under the window where she had slipped down after being the last to have the strength to lean out and try to catch a gasp of air.

All were brought down on the turntable ladder but five were already dead and the other two died shortly afterwards in hospital.

None of the women had actually been touched by flames: there was hardly a mark on them apart from smoke staining. Once more the cause of death had been the fumes. Despite the fact that they had been standing by an open window, despite the rapid reaction of the Fire Brigade, all had inhaled lethal levels of carbon monoxide fumes.

At the inquest it was made clear that the building was not a badly protected death trap and had adequate fire precautions and escapes. The initial cause of the fire remained a mystery, although an electrical fault was suspected, and the reason the victims did not get to the fire escape stayed a puzzle. The coroner, Donald Summerfield, recorded verdicts of accidental death.

If the women's first reaction on seeing the smoke had been, as we believe, not to make for the fire escape but to back away and hope for help then they would have been on the phone to the Fire Brigade instantly. The call was received at 6.48 p.m. and at that time, the evidence of the tape tells us, several if not all of the women were alive and sufficiently conscious to be shouting for help.

However, when the first fireman arrived a mere four minutes later the yelling had stopped. The women had died in that short space of time without the flames ever actually getting into the room. Eighteen children lost their mothers, not because of the intensity of the fire but through the stealth and speed of its main weapon.

The message for anyone faced with a fire, especially with one in a public place, is always the same: get out as fast as you possibly can. Leave your shopping, leave your business papers, to hell with the laptop, abandon everything and concentrate on nothing but escape. You almost certainly have less time than you think you do.

Fire kills fewer people than you might think.

The *smoke* usually gets you first.

17

Under Age

I had been warned before being ushered through the front door of a terraced home in Collyhurst Street, Collyhurst, Manchester, in the spring of 1982, that this one was pretty dreadful. It was a child again, a baby actually.

David Joynson was just four months old, a little thing, not yet crawling. He had not been long enough in the world to learn much about it. All he knew was that there were faces around him that he found reassuring. They would smile at him and give him affection and clothe him and keep him warm and feed him. The chances are that – until he died – no one had been at all unpleasant towards him.

It was easy to picture him on his back, grinning widely and waving his arms and legs in the air, seeking attention, gurgling in pleasure. He was a regular, bright kid.

No more.

He was on the settee. From his toes to the now unseeing eyes there was nothing particular to remark on. But the top of his skull had been blown away and most of his brain was spattered over the furniture. There was smoke staining and small pellet entry wounds on the right side of his head above and in front of the right ear.

My examination found that there were no other external abnormalities.

Internally he was a perfectly healthy and well-nourished baby. He had died from a shotgun blast to the head at very close range. Fragments of brain and skull were scattered all over the room, on the ceiling and on the walls but most of it did not belong to the boy.

His father's body lay at the side of the settee, face down in a pool of blood. A cartridge case was visible beside the feet of the man and when we turned him over we found the shotgun hidden underneath him.

He was wearing a white shirt, an anorak, trousers, underpants and socks. Both arms were tattooed, a ring was present on the third finger of his right hand, a medallion was on a chain around his neck and a digital watch was on his left wrist.

Much of his face and skull were missing. There was extensive destruction of the left side of his head, the left of the forehead and the nose. Smoke staining on the chin, along with the extensive destruction of the base of the skull and the hard palate in the top of the mouth, suggested emphatically that the point of entry for the shot was through the mouth. The man, like his son, was otherwise in good health and had died from a single gunshot wound to the head. The weapon in both cases was probably the twelve-bore shotgun found at the scene.

A blood-alcohol test showed 25 milligrams of alcohol per 100 millilitres of blood. Joynson Snr, a twenty-seven-year-old taxi driver, had been drunk but not to the extent that he would not have been able to think fairly rationally or reasonably control himself.

The initial impression was that the father had shot the son and then turned the weapon on himself, though, of course, everyone anticipated a lot of work was ahead to prove for sure that was what had happened. At this early stage of the investigation it was still possible to speculate that a third party might have committed a foul double murder and cunningly attempted to make it look like a murder-suicide.

In fact, from a detection point of view, it became very straightforward. The police got a confession.

One sharp-eyed officer at the scene noticed a tell-tale light on a tape recorder that indicated the machine in a corner of the room was switched on. The cassette tape in it had run its length and stopped. It was rewound, the 'play' button was punched and the last words Robert Joynson ever spoke were clearly heard by everyone.

He and his girlfriend Diane, young David's mother, had recently split up and she had taken the boy with her. He was devastated by the separation and twice took a mild overdose in an effort to engender sympathy and get her back.

But anger – fury, even – was never far removed from the debilitating sadness he felt and two days before the deaths the more destructive emotions took control. Joynson warned Diane: 'I am going to hurt you one day.'

Despite the threats Diane was reasonable about access arrangements and happy enough to leave the youngster with his father for a day. She could not have known, but that was a fatal error.

Joynson spent the day drinking and brooding and then made a monumental decision. He was clear in his boiling mind that he wanted to hurt Diane and he cared nothing for the consequences. The fact that hurting her in the most painful manner available to him would also involve hurting his own flesh and blood was something he was prepared for, but not something he could live with.

301

He turned on the tape and sealed his fate. That one, simple act ensured there was no turning back. The tape became a co-conspirator, an evil entity in itself that watched his every move. And insisted he take each damnable, irrevocable step. It was his Slavemaster.

Without the tape Joynson could always have stopped before it was too late, changed his mind, come to his senses, recanted. It would have been failure and cowardice in his own eyes, but it would not have been public. No one would have known. But by activating the machine he had a witness – and that was that. The tape was running and he had to run with it. Inexorably, it reeled him in.

Most of the message on the machine was furious drink-enhanced ranting as Joynson sought for someone to blame for what he was about to do. Then he became more clinical and described his actions.

He described David lying back on the settee, described the gun, and explained what he was doing with it, how he was pointing it at the boy and getting closer. In a direct message to Diane he said: 'If I cannot have David, you cannot either.' Then there was a loud bang followed shortly afterwards by a second. The tape then continued to run on in absolute silence. The silence went on for a long time.

With the killer dead there was no need for a trial but, at the inquest which followed, the coroner, Leonard Gorodkin, remarked: 'This is a most unusual situation in that we have an actual recording and it is clear that the baby was shot and then Mr Joynson shot himself.'

The tape was not played in court but the jury were provided with a transcript. Members of Joynson's family said they wanted to hear the tape as there might have been some information on it of some significance. But the coroner ruled against them.

He decided that while the tape was evidence and its contents should be placed before the jury it was also a message directed specifically at Diane. She was thus the sole owner and therefore the only person he could permit to have it.

Diane, sensibly in my opinion, never listened to her son die, never heard his killer's taunts and ordered the police to destroy the tape forthwith.

While Joynson got his vengeance, while he claimed, brutally and selfishly, the young life that he and Diane had created between them, Diane's wise decision ruined his final, warped intention.

He never got to mock or to gloat. He just died.

Another child who suffered at the hands of a violent father was dealt a different, but in many ways more appalling hand by fate, chance, God or whatever force it is that determines the path our lives take.

The law does not allow me to identify the family to you, so I shall call them the Joneses. Ian Jones was twelve at the time in question, January 1990. His father, Michael, was seventy, his mother, Mary, fifty-two.

It was Mary's second marriage; Michael was her former husband's former best friend. She had given up a great deal to abandon her previous family and most of her friends for Michael, a man much older than her, but she loved him with a passion she had not felt before. He was a big man, weighing in at twenty stone and toughened by a hard, outdoor life. She loved his strength.

They lived on a forty-acre farm in Haslingden, Lancashire, and like all farmers Michael worked long hours. Like many farmers, too, he was old-fashioned and expected his wife to be what he considered 'wifely' and know her place. She found it was important to have his meals on the table at a certain time, his clothes ready, the house tidy. He drank a lot. Like far too many men, when he was drunk or unhappy or both he got violent with his family.

However, unlike most men Michael's violence was laced with a genuinely wicked imagination. Once, weary of his tantrums, Mary briefly left him. But, of course, it was difficult to leave permanently: she had so few places to go.

Mary returned to face the music but this time Michael didn't beat her. This time her punishment was already in place and was much more hurtful than mere physical violence. Time is a great healer. It can help restore torn and bruised tissue and it can help a victim forget the memory of the pain. But there are some hurts nothing can diminish. Some wounds are so deep that, though they may not be fatal, they are beyond healing.

Mary loved riding: it was the thing that gave her the most joy. When riding she was free and happy. She had her pick of the horses in the farm's stables and, like all riders, she had her favourite, a tall grey. When she returned home that time she discovered that Michael had killed the horse and had its hooves fashioned into ashtrays. They were on the table.

Mary's son Ian shared two things with his mother, her love of horses and her abject fear of the ogre he knew as his father. The boy had won scores of trophies for showing horses and it was the main thing that he could concentrate on to take his mind off the thought of the next thrashing.

When Michael tired of knocking his wife unconscious, he used Ian to punish her. Each slap, punch or kick he gave the boy was much more painful to the child's mother than any blow he inflicted on her. Short of money once, he sold Ian's pet pony and spent all the cash on booze. One of the youngster's earliest memories of his father was when he ran over Ian's legs with a tractor.

More painful still was when Michael informed Ian that the boy was a bastard, that he, Michael, was not his natural father. The child was told that he was the product of his mother's sluttish behaviour with someone else. It was a lie designed purely to cause the child, not yet in his teens and desperately close to his mother, the greatest suffering possible. To this man, causing pain had become so strong a habit that you cannot help but wonder whether he might have somehow been addicted to it.

When the latest routine beating was over Ian would retire to his room and cry. His mother never remembered him ever attempting to fight back or shout at his father in a threatening manner. There was no point.

Then, one winter's day, after another thrashing for them both, the chubby-faced child, just six and a half stone, turned to Mary with a look in his eye that she had never seen before. He told her: 'I can't take it any more. One day I'm going to kill him.'

The coldness of the stare told her more than the words. Despite Ian's tender years, though his voice was yet to break, Mary recognized a savage maturity in his glance and immediately took him seriously. While most mothers might have just told him to forget such a silly idea, she pleaded with him not to be rash. She cared nothing any more for her husband's life but she realized the grave risk to them both. There was never any thought of getting away with it. She knew for sure that if her son carried out his threat the boy would be taken away from her, and that was far too high a price for her freedom.

The following day Ian was late home from school. Did he do it on purpose, or was it fate? I don't know, but it was no surprise to anyone that it infuriated Michael Jones. The ageing, angry bully ranted, raved and swore at the boy who bent his head in supplication and walked upstairs to his room.

An hour later the boy came back down the stairs and his father started raving once more. Ian simply turned his back and returned to the first-floor landing. This time he went not to his own room but to another, where he knew there was a shotgun. He lived on a farm, he knew how to load the gun and how to remove the safety catch. He knew how to hold it, how to point it and how to squeeze the trigger. It was too big for him but he'd been brought up tough and he gritted his teeth with the effort.

The twelve-year-old boy who two hours earlier had been with his classmates talking about football, who had not yet had a girlfriend, who had not yet tried to shave, stood four steps from the bottom of the staircase in the kitchen. With tears rolling down his cheeks, he levelled the single-barrelled weapon at his father.

Michael's reaction was typical and fatal. Instead of for once in his life backing down, instead of treating his son with some respect for no better reason than that, for once, the child had a power advantage, instead of seeing sense, the farmer strode forwards like a belligerent bull.

His last words were: 'Don't point that at me, you little bastard.'

When I arrived at the farm at 6.12 p.m. I was shown the body of an adult male lying face upwards with the arms and legs outstretched, bloodstaining on the clothing at the front and blood escaping from the mouth. The corpse was taken to Rossendale public mortuary where, at 7.50 p.m., I began the post-mortem.

He was well built, five feet ten and fully clothed. On the right side of the chest, four feet, five inches from the heel, was an area five inches square that showed multiple pellet wounds. I counted fifty-eight separate small wounds, with a single main wound in the centre about half an inch in diameter. The skull and meninges were healthy and the brain showed some small areas of old softening.

The trachea and bronchi contained blood and the lungs had pellet holes in the right upper and middle lobes, with extensive haemhorrage in this area. The left lung contained inhaled blood. Blood and blood clot were present in the right pleural cavity.

There was extensive bruising involving the muscle over the base of the right chest and two pellets were removed from there. The intercostal spaces between the second and third ribs and the third and fourth were lacerated and the right second rib was fractured.

The heart was enlarged due to hypertrophy of the left ventricle and there was blood in the pericardial sac. Two pellets were lying on the surface of the heart but had not penetrated through into the chambers. The coronary arteries showed moderate atheroma and the aorta and major vessels showed severe arteriosclerosis. The ascending aorta had multiple pellet wounds with haemorrhage along the lining of the blood vessel that extended into the pericardial sac.

The kidneys showed severe nephrosclerosis, indicating a long history of alcohol intake but the ureters, bladder and generative organs were all healthy.

Death had been caused by a single gunshot wound to the chest consistent with a single cartridge fired from a shotgun.

The position of the body and the condition of the injury coincided with everything that Ian Jones and his mother told the police. Further inquiries confirmed the husband and father had a history of drinking and violence.

In court the little boy pleaded guilty to murder and was placed in care indefinitely. He wasn't suspected of being a danger to others but to release him immediately on a guilty plea to murder is not possible under British law. Further, there was no doubt that the experience of living with such a monster and then killing him had been traumatic in the extreme and would most likely have brought any young person to the end of their emotional tether. He needed help. He needed time.

After the case was heard at Preston Crown Court, Mary remembered the moment of death and spoke of Ian.

'He just looked at me with the gun still in his hand and said: "We're free now, Mum. He can't hurt you any more." And we were free, I've never felt anything like it in my life. Ian's father, the man I had lived with for twenty-one years, was lying dead on the floor and all we felt was relief.'

One hopes that by now this mother and son who had suffered so much are reunited.

18

Making Faces

Had he been standing, the man would have looked like someone to avoid. He was in a threatening, aggressive position, his fists clenched, his arms up in a boxer's stance, his legs slightly bent as if to lower his centre of gravity to achieve better balance.

As it was, he was lying on his back, adopting what is known within forensic pathology as the 'pugilistic attitude'.

This occurs when there is a coagulation of the muscle protein due to being exposed to extreme heat. The muscles tighten, causing the joints to flex, the knees and elbows to bend. Of course, a person needs to be dead for this to happen, as was the case here for a man with no name and no face.

The fire caused by the petrol thrown over his prone body had charred or burned off more than eighty per cent of his skin. The only areas not burned were a section on his back that had been protected by the damp ground on which he lay and two narrow strips on his face, apparently shielded from the worst of the heat by a blindfold and a gag. The rest had gone.

The victim had been found, still smouldering, at three a.m. on Saturday, 19 March 1988. At six a.m., in the company of Detective Chief Superintendent Roy Fletcher of Lancashire CID, I was taken to view the remains lying close to a gateway that led to Dean Clough reservoir, Blackburn Old Road, Great Harwood, near Accrington. An hour later I started my examination at Blackburn Royal Infirmary.

The subject was five feet, three inches tall and had all his thirty-two teeth, weighed eleven stone and had been circumcised. The intense burning had left only scanty remains of clothing and the heat had split the skin on the arms, chest and legs.

Around the neck were strands of three-core electric cable with the plastic cover burned away and the metal wires fused together. It had been tightly applied.

There were two areas of less burned skin on the face. The first, which went across the mouth and the right side of the face, was one inch wide. The second, slightly narrower, could be traced across the right eye. The two converged at a point just below the lower lobe of the right ear. The shape suggested a gag and blindfold having been in position, each tied behind the head.

Externally, there were two lacerations to the head, one two inches long to the back left side and the other, half an inch long, above the outer part of the left eyebrow. There was also a bruise to the left side of the upper lip.

Internally there was bruising beneath both external head wounds and bruising on the left side of the chest corresponding with a fracture of the eighth rib on the left side.

However, there was also a depressed fracture of the skull near the temple that did not correspond to any appreciable external damage but did match with diffuse bruising of the cerebral hemispheres of the brain and the tip of the temporal lobe. Death had occurred as a result of cerebral haemorrhage caused by this fracture of the skull.

If, as seems likely, the fatal blow was the final blow of the assault, the lack of external bruising could be explained in one of two ways. Either death occurred rapidly, before signs of bruising (caused by blood flow) could develop, or the victim had already been in a deep state of shock from the earlier stages of the attack, which caused his circulation to be sluggish and unable to deliver the blood to the affected area before the heart ceased to function.

There was no carbon dioxide in the blood and no signs of inhaled smoke, indicating that he had been dead before his body was set alight.

Despite the ferocity of the blaze and its destructive power, much had been learned about this anonymous man and the manner of his passing.

The cause of his death was a blow to the head with a blunt instrument, probably one of three such blows. There were no defence wounds on the hands or forearms, suggesting he was either taken by surprise or not in a position to defend himself when the final assault came.

The lip bruising could have been caused by a blow to the mouth or by pressure caused by a tight ligature. If it was the latter then the bruising would prove he was alive when it was applied.

The chest injuries were consistent with a heavy fall.

The pugilistic attitude suggested that he was laid out straight when the fire began, which in turn meant that the chances were that the assault did not take place where he was burned. One does not usually 'lay out' someone immediately after a battle that is to end with cremation. More likely the victim was transported to this place after death and the rib damage could have been caused when he was being placed in a car boot or being pulled from it.

313

The apparent gag and blindfold marks could equally have been caused by a ligature holding in place a hood, perhaps to prevent blood or vomit from staining the transport. While the injuries found around the neck could have been an attempt at strangulation there were no signs on the body – such as larynx damage or petechial haemorrhages – to suggest it had been even partially successful. Again, it could have been part of the tying-up process after death.

The extent of the pugilistic attitude told us that he had been burned before rigor mortis had set in, probably within two hours of his death. Post-rigor, the posture would have been more exaggerated. Further, as there was little sign of decomposition, it was unlikely that sufficient time had elapsed between death and burning for rigor to have come and gone.

What little skin remained was the dark shade of an Asian but quite hairy, so probably not a Japanese or Chinese. If he was Asian then the circumcision suggested he may have been of the Muslim faith.

His round face, squat nose with a wide bridge (the shape was still clear even without skin), and straight hair also suggested Asian origins.

So we knew a fair deal about the cause of death and the victim's likely general origins, which was extremely interesting from my point of view. But for the murder-inquiry detectives it was, at best, disappointingly limited. However, that terribly damaged face with all but its most basic features obliterated was soon to offer much more concrete information.

Det Chief Supt Fletcher now had some insight into what had happened and tended to lean away from any gangland-crime motive. Hit men, even those choosing blunt instruments as their method of dispatch, tend to use much more force than this. Of three blows only one split the skull. There was no overkill, none of the 'let's make certain' attitude of the hired killer.

This was probably the work of someone not used to dishing out violent punishment. It could well have been a domestic matter.

Further, it seemed that the killer or killers believed that the mere identification of the victim would bring the police to their door. This was why they had attempted to incinerate the body to such an extent that it could never be recognized. The burning, they hoped, would obliterate their victim's features and fingerprints and ruin any chance of him being identified.

After a second post-mortem that confirmed my findings, the hands were removed and sent to a forensic laboratory where attempts were made to get even a partial print. The head was severed and taken to Manchester University.

Richard Neave, an artist whose primary duty there is to produce phenomenally detailed illustrations for medical textbooks, has an unusual extra string to his bow. He is probably the world's leading authority in the art of facial reconstruction.

Back in 1973 he was invited to put faces to two Egyptian mummies unwrapped at Manchester Museum. Later, archaeologists asked him to work on the visages of no lesser luminaries than Philip of Macedon (the father of Alexander the Great) and King Midas, noted for his touch.

Famously, the artist recreated the features of a 2,000-year-old murder victim found buried in peat at Lindow Common, Wilmslow, Cheshire. Naturally the body was named Lindow Pete.

Here, faced with a modern murder, Neave studied the head of the man with no name and took photographs from every conceivable angle. There was little left to the untrained eye but, nevertheless, that which remained was significant and was to assist considerably the accuracy of his reconstruction. The head was still its original shape, not squashed by time underground and not missing sections, and the shape of the nose was quite clear, a detail which a decomposed body would fail to provide.

But to get close to the exact shape of the facial bones Neave needed to get down to the skull, so the skin had to be removed completely. (Hence the second post-mortem: there was no going back.)

After this a cast replica of the skull was made, which allowed the original to be returned to the police and reunited with its torso for eventual burial or cremation, this time of an official nature.

Neave began by drilling tiny holes at twenty-one strategic points on the replica skull – on the temple, forehead, lips, jaw and chin – and inserted a cocktail stick in each. This formed his matrix and made possible the pinpoint precision necessary as he delicately applied clay to build up the soft tissue in varying depths and shapes over the blank skull.

The contours of the skull and the positions of the eyes, nose and mouth and the spaces between them all have a known relationship with the soft tissues of the face that sit upon this specific shape. Each detail is worked out from a set of established measurements that state the precise depth of tissue at any single key point on the face to the nearest hundredth of a millimetre.

Using his vast knowledge of facial anatomy (and with a detailed reference book at his side) Neave worked to add first the muscles that lie over the jaw, cheeks and forehead, knowing where each would be attached, its length and width and its direction.

Age, race and sex are all factors and he was able to use his knowledge that this was probably an Asian male aged between thirty and fifty.

So the skin was .75 millimetres thicker over the eyebrow than over the forehead but nearly double that at the lower lip – and so on. Each tiny embellishment – based on science but with the touch of an artist – added a little more to the whole.

The shape of the lips, though, had to be a matter of educated conjecture as the skull cannot determine that feature. Similarly with the eyelids, although here again the likelihood of an Asian origin for the victim helped.

When finished, the face still had a stark 'deadness' to it. But a gentle softening of the edges suggested the elasticity of real skin and a small round hole in the centre of the eyes gave it 'life'. Neave knew the victim did not have a squint as the eyes were not burned, and his last act, to create their pupils and in them the impression of awareness, of living, awakened the face as if from a trance.

The likeness was to prove so remarkable that Neave was later to describe the work he did on the skull of Sabbir Kassam Kilu as his greatest forensic triumph.

The face appeared on TV and was instantly recognized as that of a thirty-eight-year-old property developer from Leicester who had vanished four weeks previously.

The detective had been right. The act of identifying the man led straight to his killers. Mr Kilu's wife, her brother and her sister were all found guilty of murder at Liverpool Crown Court.

In evidence the brother claimed that Kilu had raped his sister-in-law at his home and she had hit him over the head with a masala (a wooden herb-crusher similar to a rounders bat). This was consistent with the head injury discovered at the post-mortem.

He added that the body had been wrapped in a blanket that had been securely tied – again, consistent with the apparent blindfold and gag marks found on his face.

He also stated that his sister put a wire around the dead man's neck in order to lift him up. Once more the story tallied with the findings.

They drove the corpse of Sabbir Kilu north, dumped it at a secluded spot and set it alight. On the way back to Leicester they would confidently have believed that the flames they had left burning were consuming the evidence against them.

Without the unusual skill of Richard Neave, the man who makes faces, they might have been right.

19

The Empty Sport

Although one should always go into any pathological examination with a completely open mind, it is often impossible not to have at least some preconceived idea about what killed someone.

You always have some information about the patient available, whether it is a case of an apparent heart attack, kidney failure or a gunshot wound to the chest, and you automatically look for those things that will confirm the pre-investigative diagnosis.

More often than not, my job entailed confirming to people what they thought had happened, although there were several occasions when the cause of death was eventually discovered to differ from everyone's expectations.

However, it was most unusual for me to be instantly surprised by what I found when I opened someone up. Such was the case back in the late 1950s when we had a look at a boxer called Jackie Tiller.

He had been an amateur fighter while serving in the Army. But, by all accounts, he wasn't that accomplished because he was discharged with some form of brain damage and advised to give up the sport for good.

Sadly, boxing was all Jackie knew. Faced with a choice, as he saw it, between starving or fighting, he kept his gloves on and joined a touring professional boxing booth, taking on all comers.

I'm not sure how much success Jackie had or over what period of time. But his last fight was at Doncaster when a local bruiser caught him with a big right and he hit the canvas hard.

He was taken unconscious to the neurosurgical unit at Sheffield where he remained in a coma for several months. His family was based in Manchester and eventually he was transferred to the city's Withington Hospital where, after a few more weeks of unconsciousness, he died.

I anticipated that his final demise had been brought on by bronchial pneumonia. That's normally the case with long-term coma patients who have been on life-support machines. Their respiratory systems become deeply depressed, having not been able to function unaided for such a long period, and their bodies finally become immune to the antibiotics they are being given to keep infection at bay.

What we found in his chest was certainly in line with what we expected. But it was what we found – or did not find – in his skull that was so remarkable.

Jackie Tiller had no brain.

The membranes that surround the grey matter were still there. But inside them, instead of the familiar rounded, knobbly shape of the brain, was clear liquid, no more viscous than water. It was, to all intents and purposes, a water-filled balloon with as much chance of creating thought as a Party Popper.

In his life the boxer had often been knocked senseless. But the last blow he received was to leave him brainless.

In what was one of the first serious medical examinations

connected with the sport of boxing, my colleagues and I considered carefully what we knew about Jackie's lifestyle. We analysed the punishment he was likely to receive in a day or week and utilized this in our investigations into how his brain came to be in such a state.

Normally the brain breathes because blood circulates within it through the ventricles, much like any other organ. Oxygenated blood penetrates the brain itself and then passes through tiny holes or granulations that form over the outer surface before being delivered back down the spinal cord and returning through the circulatory system to the heart where it is pumped around again.

The brain is surrounded by a membrane that is itself suspended in a liquid solution that in turn is held inside the skull. The liquid absorbs the everyday shocks of movement and can handle such matters as running, jumping or heading a modern light football with relative ease.

But sudden, rapid movement can generate sufficient force to push the liquid aside and bang the brain against the side of the skull. Further, a direct blow, particularly to the chin, can send a shock up through the jaw that can then slam against the base of the brain.

When such violence occurs it is not unusual for small haemorrhages to be caused. We eventually came to the conclusion that they had formed scar tissue that had blocked up the granulations. This prevented the blood filtrate escaping from within the brain, and filled it up from the inside to develop an advanced state of hydrocephalus with pressure so strong that it was sufficient, over time, to compress the brain away.

Jackie survived with the aid of machines because our automatic functions are handled by the brain stem or mid-brain. With such help, he could breathe and his heart would beat. But nothing could have helped him to think.

This case led me inescapably to the conclusion that boxing is a barbaric sport and should have no place in civilized society.

It is the only sport where the object is to do enough damage to the head of an opponent to render him (or her, nowadays, I am appalled to say) unconscious. Other contact sports involve making the other person incapable of attacking, but boxing has captured the deliberate-head-injury market.

My mind wasn't changed by the case of a fifteen-year-old boy who was part of the boxing entertainment at a Sportsman's Dinner in Saddleworth, near Oldham. The fight was recorded on video by a doctor who was a guest at the event.

Viewing it later, it was clear that the bout was badly mismatched and the boy was getting a heavy beating from a bigger fighter. The video also showed to my satisfaction that it was poorly refereed and should have been stopped before it was finished by yet another heavy blow to the boy's head.

He collapsed in one of the corners of the boxing ring and died very quickly. He had suffered a massive clot over the surface of the brain, which is invariably fatal unless treated expertly within minutes.

Professional bouts have specialist doctors available ring-side who are aware of what signs to look for and have the know-how to handle such a situation. Even then, the chances of survival are slim. But in this case, at a low-key junior amateurs fight, there was no such luxury.

In a young boy, the brain is large relative to the size of the skull. So a tear inside the brain, as in this case, causing blood to rush out and fill the space within the skull, would, crucially, bring about death quicker than in an adult.

It is the sort of injury I also see when drunks fall over and hit the pavement, or when tiny babies have been powerfully shaken from side to side.

Since that fight, protective headgear has been made compulsory at amateur matches. There is also a greater awareness now of the damage that can be done even if the combatants are only fighting over three rounds.

It is not just the sudden deaths that make the sport of boxing unacceptable: there is overwhelming evidence of serious long-term injury. The simple fact is that men who box will often die ten or twenty years earlier than they should because of the damage the 'Noble Sport' did to them when they were younger.

You only have to look at the terrible way that boxing's greatest-ever ambassador, Muhammad Ali, has declined from wisecracking, handsome superman to the sad, shuffling, incoherent individual he is now to realize the effects such unremitting punishment can have.

All right, he is ill for other reasons as well, according to people close to him. But no one can tell me that being hit didn't play a major role in his physical and mental decline. Admittedly he was hit by experts, from Smokin' Joe Frazier to big George Foreman before he got fat, but it only needs one blow to land wrong and anyone can be permanently damaged.

In a perfect world I'd ban the game. But that would probably only drive it underground and back to the bare fists.

Further, one has to accept the rights of people to choose whether or not to get involved in such a thing. One must retain liberty even if it means allowing people to take foolish, unnecessary risks as a result of which their brains can be literally reduced to mush.

Having said that, how many of us now regret the seat-belt law or the law about the wearing of motorcycle helmets? At first they met opposition from the freedom lobby but the statistics have since proved that they save lives.

Today, anyone who doesn't 'belt up' or wear a helmet is considered to be a halfwit.

Mind you, that's fifty per cent better than poor Jackie Tiller.

20

The Lord of Strangeways

The day I quit I helped a killer get off. I knew he was a killer – I'd helped put him away in the first place. It was a strange way of ending a career, in more ways than one.

Alan Lord was a brute. He may still be. A gargantuan, hugely powerful man, he ran with gangs, enjoyed pushing his considerable weight around and liked the idea that people feared him.

No doubt he was filled with insecurities going right back to a difficult and possibly unhappy childhood and had developed a massive physique to give him a presence he never had as a troubled adolescent and teenager. This was his way of handling his own special demons.

So much for the excuses.

He was also an unpleasant yob who, at the age of twenty, led a small group who viciously attacked and robbed a talented jazz musician.

David Gilbert was by night a saxophonist and clarinettist with the Delta Jazz Band and by day made a living working for a jeweller, mending timepieces. He was a quiet, unassuming and peaceful individual who had spent five years at the Royal Manchester College of Music, desperately wanted to play for a living, but had been disappointed by the harsh realities of the music-business world.

One snowy night in January 1981 the thirty-six-year-old

father of three was unfortunate enough to be walking home with his briefcase when he was spotted by Lord and his cronies who had set out to commit a robbery. Their intended victim was the manager of a furniture shop but, employing the consummate tactical planning of professional criminals, they arrived only to discover he had locked up and gone home.

Thwarted but still hyped up, they cast around for another victim and found him in the slight form of Mr Gilbert. They caught him in a footpath between Bury Old Road and Polygon Road, Crumpsall, Manchester, and stole his case containing twelve watches, watchmaking equipment and a hairbrush. They cruelly left him to die where he fell.

It was 8.45 p.m. on Thursday, 16 January and very cold when I arrived at the murder scene. The victim was lying face upwards next to a fence. A mouthpiece was in place, having been used by an ambulance crew in an effort at resuscitation. Blood was on the front of the clothing and down the trousers.

A little over an hour later, at the Manchester central mortuary, we checked the victim's clothes: a jacket, green polo-neck sweater, grey trousers, underpants, socks and shoes.

My notes show there was a scrape mark on the front of the right ankle, bruising on the base of the right index finger, abrasions on the knuckles of the right hand between the little and ring fingers and at the base of the middle finger.

There was an abrasion on the right side of the chin, bruising on the right cheek and right side of the face and an abrasion on the right side of the forehead. There was a scratch mark on the right side of the neck sixteen centimetres long, running from the larynx to the right ear which was consistent with a slashing wound from a knife.

In the midline of the chest at the lower end of the breast bone was a stab wound twelve millimetres long (I had finally capitulated and moved on to metric.) There was a small abrasion on the right buttock and a stab wound fifteen millimetres long in the back.

The wound to the front of the chest had pierced the sternum at the junction of the fourth and fifth ribs with the breast bone. There was extensive blood clot in the anterior mediastinum.

There was blood and an incised laceration in the right side of the pericardial sac that entered the right ventricle, pierced the septum of the heart and entered the left ventricle.

The left lung was healthy but the right lung showed a stab wound that had entered the lower lobe for about two centimetres and had caused haemorrhage into the surrounding lung tissue. There was further haemorrhage in the right pleural cavity and we collected around two pints of blood. The rear of the thoracic cavity had been penetrated, the injury entering the chest at the level of the eighth rib and passing close to the spine.

The deceased had suffered two penetrating wounds to the chest, one at the front and one at the back. Each had penetrated into the body cavity for about three and a half inches (so much for metric), the one at the front penetrating the heart and the one at the back piercing the lung. Either of these wounds could have proved fatal on their own. He had died of haemorrhage caused by stab wounds to the chest.

Later I was shown a knife with a four-inch blade. I told

the police it was capable of causing the injuries I had seen. It was Lord's knife.

After his so-called pals put him in the frame, the jury at Manchester Crown Court took little time to convict him. Mr Justice Russell told him: 'You killed this man with the utmost ferocity. It is a dreadful case.' Lord got life.

While it was a dreadful murder it was hardly a spectacular case, compared to many. The murderer would probably have been forgotten by now by all but his own family – and his victim's – had it not been for the Strangeways riot.

On All Fools Day, 1990, the inmates at Manchester's jail took over the complex and began its systematic destruction. The reasons why it happened are many and complex, but the immediate consequences were very simple and straightforward.

On the first two days that the men had control, a great deal of anger overflowed among the violent and the wretched. The prisoners felt a sense of freedom but they were still incarcerated, still behind the big wall. Lord and others smashed their way through the roof and sat on the tiles, waving at the Press and hurling missiles uselessly at the riot shields below. They were on top of the world, out in the sunshine, and still as much prisoners as they had ever been.

They were going nowhere. Angrily they turned their attention to the 'nonces' or 'beasts', those either convicted or accused of sex crimes who, under Rule 43 of the prison system, were segregated from the rest on E Wing for their own protection.

One such man was remand prisoner and father-to-be Derek White, aged forty-seven. His blood was spattered five feet up his cell walls. He was savagely beaten, thrown off a landing into a 'suicide' safety net, possibly twice, and

328

suffered dreadfully for several hours. He was rescued from the jail by prison staff and was able to walk, with assistance, from the prison to an ambulance that took him to hospital. Initially he seemed not to have any life-threatening injuries but, suddenly, he died.

It was clear from the first time I saw White that he had taken a terrible beating. There were bruises around the right elbow, the right wrist, the back of the left arm, the front of the chest, around the right eye, over both shoulders and in the left groin. The right shoulder had been dislocated and there was a laceration in the eyebrow that had been sutured.

The scalp showed extensive bruising on the left side but the skull was intact and the brain was healthy. The lungs were congested and there was extensive bruising posterially in the left pleural cavity.

There was a fracture of the fifth rib at its junction with the sternum on the left side but this appeared to have been caused during attempts at resuscitation. On the right side there was extensive bruising of the lower ribs with small crack fractures of the sixth and seventh ribs.

The heart was normal but the pulmonary artery on each side contained numerous ante-mortem thrombi consistent with having originated in deep veins.

While White's injuries were extensive they would not have killed him. He was the victim of a pulmonary embolism caused by a thrombosis (blood clot) that had formed elsewhere in his body, travelled to the heart and brought about his sudden death. Such a thrombosis could be caused by a severe blow, for instance the sort of trauma one might suffer if hit several times by a bunch of half-crazy prisoners during a riot.

A later dissection by another pathologist revealed a one-inch-diameter bruise at the back of the right leg above the ankle. This was where the fatal thrombosis had begun.

It was a reasonable assumption that Mr White's death had been caused by the rioters. The ringleaders of the riot were known. This was a very high-profile case. Five, including Lord, were charged with murder but the prosecution never had a chance of getting a guilty verdict. Although they knew that, they allowed the case to go on for thirty days before I was called to ruin things. I had told them the problems, informed them the case was unwinnable, so I can only imagine the politicians wanted the publicity.

If publicity was needed, Alan Lord provided it two months after coming down off the prison roof. As the jail was no longer fit for habitation, inmates were farmed out to police stations. Lord, being a ringleader and a lifer, was placed in the most secure in Greater Manchester, at Astley Bridge in Bolton. Absurdly, he found a bunch of keys and escaped.

Dubbed 'Britain's most wanted man', he was traced to a house in Liverpool five days later but still nearly gave his pursuers the slip. He heard them coming and left the house without using a door. He threw his giant frame through a French window and ran straight through the window of a neighbour's house, then through another – and another.

Finally, the police caught up with Lord and he pretended, badly cut from his efforts, to be dead. He was working on the possibility that they might just leave him where he was until an undertaker arrived, so giving him another chance to run. The police handcuffed the 'corpse' by both wrists and both ankles, just in case.

Preposterously, three years later, while the massive trial

resulting from the Strangeways riot was still under way, Lord did it again. Few men have ever embarrassed the system as much as Alan Lord did.

This time he and four others broke into the ceiling space in the room where they were being held in the basement of the Manchester Crown Court building. They managed to crawl through to Court 2, dropped down and walked into a hallway.

When they stepped out of the court they were shocked to see a senior judge walking towards them. Perhaps fortunately for him he failed to recognize them, assumed they were workmen, and was happy to give them directions to the nearest exit.

They were all recaptured within a matter of weeks, Lord after seventeen days and while making a call from a public phone in Ordsall, Salford. You would have thought that if he had really wanted to stay out of prison he would this time have got well clear of the North West of England.

The likely truth is that outside jail Alan Lord wasn't much to be reckoned with, despite his bulk and penchant for violence, while inside he was a Main Man. He was most probably quite relieved to be heading home.

While Lord was on the run this second time, he and the others charged with Derek White's murder got a boost from me.

I was called to give evidence and the prosecution asked me all the right questions. I explained to the jury that the embolism that killed White could have been caused by the dreadful beating he received at the hands of the prison inmates during the riot. Then, of course, the defence stood up.

I knew what they were going to ask. Could I be absolutely

sure that the embolism was caused during the riot? The answer: 'No.'

Was it possible that the embolism had been caused by some other means and at some other time? The answer was an impossible-to-avoid 'Yes'. Yes, Derek White might not have died as a direct result of the injuries received during the riot. It was a possibility I could not rule out. There was reasonable doubt.

This was not just my opinion. Several other pathologists' opinions on the subject were heard by the court and all came to the same conclusion. It was impossible to be certain when the fatal blood clot had formed.

This could not have come as a surprise to the prosecution as it was something that had been discussed at length previously. But at least they had taken full advantage of their thirty days of evidence to show the public where authority really lies in this country.

Mr Justice Mantell instructed the jury to find the five formally not guilty of murder. The trial for riot continued and Lord was eventually found guilty and sentenced to ten years in prison – on top of his life sentence for the murder of Mr Gilbert. He wasn't in court to hear the sentence passed down – he was still on the run after his second escape.

The police were displeased with me after my evidence. I think they had hoped I might bend a little in their direction, bearing in mind the gravity of the case. But, by the nature of my job, *all* my cases were grave, if you will pardon the pun.

I wasn't there to decide if Alan Lord was a murderer this time or the last time, to worry about what he might do next, to make a moral judgement. I wasn't there to mete out justice. I wasn't there for retribution.

My task – as always – did not involve the survivors on

either side of the law. My evidence was uncluttered by the complexities of life and the convolutions of the living.

This was my last case and, as in all the others that preceded it, I was qualified to offer an opinion on one thing and one thing only.

The cause of death.

Index

'G.M.' indicates Greater Manchester

Abortion Law Reform Act (1968)   152, 153
Abortion Law Reform Association   152
abortions   151–8
Adams, Warren   245–6
Akram, Mohammed   260
Akram, Tahir   257–8
Alexander, Kenneth   186–7
Ali, Muhammad   323
Allman, Amanda Jane   199, 200, 202–8
Allman, Darrell   207
Allman, Natalie   207
Almond River, Scotland   89
Altrincham, G.M.   93
Anderton, James (later Sir James)   117, 119
Andrew (son of Maureen Bradbury)   51, 62, 67, 68, 69
animals, death of   99–100
Ansari, Mohammed Sarwar   261–3
appeals   187–8
Ardwick, Manchester   261
Arrowe Park Hospital, Birkenhead   218
Ashton, Marie   228–30
Ashton-under-Lyne, G.M.   202, 207, 231
Ashworth, Alice   159–60
Ashworth, Mr   160
Ashworth Hospital, Merseyside   15, 18
Astley Bridge police station, Bolton   330
Atlanta, Georgia   152
Audenshaw, G.M.   259
Australian police   86

Bagley, Wythenshawe   110

Baker, Dr Stephen   286
Barnes, Martin   128–9
Barrow-in-Furness, Cumbria   126
   mortuary   126
   police station   128
Bath   165
Beardow, Sandra Elaine   154–5
Bebington, Merseyside   217
Beech, Alec   69
Beech, Demrhys (Debbie)   70, 72–7
Beech, John   70, 71–2, 74, 76
Beech, Kelly   70, 71, 76
Beech, Roy   69–71, 73–7
Beech, Samantha Jane   70, 71, 74, 75, 76
Beeson, Dr Brian   81
Bennett, Keith   13, 16, 17, 18, 185
Benstead, Dr John   286
Beswick, G.M.   238
Bidston Hill, near Birkenhead   221
Big Western pub, Moss Side, Manchester   237
Biggs, Jim   193, 194
Birch service station, near Bury, Lancashire   111
Birkenhead, Merseyside   216, 220, 221
Birmingham Six   286
Blackburn, Lancashire   227, 228
Blackburn Royal Infirmary   312
Blackley, Manchester   226
Bloods (Los Angeles gang)   172
'Blues', Moss Side, Manchester   181
Bolton, Lancashire   95, 96, 330
Bolton and District General Hospital   mortuary   117, 266
Bolton police station   265, 266
Bosnia   151
Bowden, Sergeant Jim   112–13

335

boxing 319–24
Bradbury, Alison 51, 62, 67, 68
Bradbury, Arthur 50–55, 57, 58, 62–9
Bradbury, Maureen 51–5, 58, 59, 62–8
Brady, Ian 12–19, 26, 132–3, 185
brain 97–101, 209–10
Bridge Inn, Gorton 196
Bridgewood, Lesley Sharon 207, 212
Bridgford, J.R. (estate agents, Prestbury)
    272
British Aerospace plant, Preston 188
British Army 194, 195
British Medical Association 153
Brixton, south London 167
Brown, Cecil 'Hovis' 243–6
Brown, Mrs Lesley 105
Brown, Louise 102, 105
Brownhill, Stuart 222, 225–6
Burnage, G.M. 262
Burnley mortuary 246
Butcher, Chief Superintendent 146

Callan, Kevin John 199–202, 206–13
Callow, Henry 287
Cantley, Mr Justice 249, 287
Carrington, G.M. 24
Catholic Church 104, 151
Caulfield, Mr Justice 190
Chadderton, 'Chattie' Ann 231–2
Cheetham Hill mob, Manchester 183,
    184
Cheshire police 250, 279–80
Chester Assizes 14
Chester Crown Court 156
Chicago 170, 172, 177
Chorley, Lancashire 83, 87, 90, 122, 217
Chorley Sewage Works 123
Chorlton-cum-Hardy, G.M. 181
Civil Aviation Authority 41
Clarke, Norman 235–9, 246
Clatterbridge Hospital, Wirral 95
Clift, Dr Alan 270, 271
Codling, Inspector Ray 109, 111–15,
    125
Collyhurst, Manchester 299
Cookham Wood prison, Kent 15
Court of Appeal 200–202
Craig, Clovis O'Neil 247–9
Crewe, Cheshire 250, 251
Crewe police station 250
Crighton, Mr Justice 155
crime scene
    position of the body 2

removal of the body 2
    sealed 2, 279
Crips (Los Angeles gang) 172
Crown Hotel, Birkenhead 216
Crown Prosecution Service 211
Crumpsall, Manchester 326

Dada, Mrs 263
Dada, Siddik 261, 262, 263
Data Reference Centre, Belfast 197
Davenport, Mrs 122
Davenport, PC Ray 120–22, 125
de Kretsel, Dr Dan 36
death
    of animals 99–100
    cause of 96–8
    the moment of 97–8
decomposition 94
Delta Jazz Band 325
Detroit 170, 172, 177
Diane (David Joynson's mother) 301,
    302, 303
Diggle, near Saddleworth 110
Dodd, Jack Groombridge 126–8
Doddington gang (Moss Side) 173, 174
domestic murder 44–6
Douglas Corporation 284
Downey, Christopher 7, 193–8
Downey, Lesley Ann 13–16, 23
Dr Kershaw's Cottage Hospital, Royton,
    Oldham 105
Driver, Beverley 135–6
drugs 81, 83–91, 172–9, 181–3, 259,
    261
Dunblane, Scotland 255
Dynamic Plastics 116

Edge, Arthur 116, 118–19, 122
Edwards, Bob 103, 104, 106
Egerton, PC John 116–19, 125
Enville Street Social Club, Ashton-under-
    Lyne 54
Evans, Edward 13

Failsworth, near Oldham 144
Fallowfield, Manchester 185
Farnworth, Bolton 116, 266, 269
Farquharson, Mr Justice 119
Farrow, Sheilagh 133, 140, 141–2,
    144–7
Fleming, Edward 227, 228, 230–31
Fletcher, Detective Chief Superintendent
    Roy 311, 314

Index

Flight KT 328 disaster (Manchester Airport)   29–41, 281
Foreman, George   323
Foster, Gerald   241–3
Frazier, Smokin' Joe   323
Freeman, Dr (consultant paediatrician)   202, 203, 205
Fritters nightclub, Oldham   222

Gaffey, Detective Superintendent Ron   237
Galbestos   283
Gamett, John   54, 67
gang culture
  case studies   178–91
  Jamaica   172, 173
  Manchester   173–7
  United States   172
Gardner, Anthony 'Scratch'   181–2, 183, 190
Garrett, Dr Geoffrey
  autopsy statistics   x
  consultancy at the Oldham group of hospitals   96
  first callout as Home Office pathologist   viii–x
  first job as pathologist (Bolton)   95–6
  involvement in 'test-tube' baby breakthrough   102–4, 158
  last case   325–33
  National Service   96
  Northern Nigeria post   96
  works in Casualty at Altrincham   93
Gee, Dr David   22
Gibson, Annie   195, 196
Gibson, Edward   195
Gilbert, David   325–7, 332
Girlwood barracks   194
Gooch gang (Moss Side)   173, 174
Gorodkin, Leonard   36, 237–8, 302–3
Gorton, Manchester   10, 12
Great Harwood, near Accrington   312
Greater London   256
Greater Manchester
  'bumper year' for murders (1991)   235
  racist attacks record   256
Greater Manchester CID   13
Greater Manchester Police   176, 185
  motorway section   111
Green, Alan, QC   17
Green, Dr (now Professor) Michael   22, 23, 24, 27, 206, 210, 211–12

guns
  carried by police   107–8
  dangers of a gun culture   107–8, 185, 187, 190–91
  in a drug culture   174–7

Haigh, Detective Chief Inspector Kevin   176
Hamilton, Thomas   255
Hammett, Jean   154
Hardy, Colin   142, 143, 149
Hardy, PC Justin   279–80
Hardy, Trevor Joseph   133–49, 215, 222
Harpurhey, Greater Manchester   51, 140
Harrison, Kristina   111
Harrison, Melvyn   269–71
Haslingden, Lancashire   304
Hattersley, Cheshire   13
Hazel Grove, Stockport   110
heart function   97, 98–9
Heath, Neville   141
Hennegan, Ann   55, 57, 58, 60–61, 62, 64, 67, 68, 69
Hennegan, Mr   55
Henriques, Mr Richard, QC   202
Heskin Delph, near Chorley   81
Hill, Wing Commander Ian   40
Hindley, Myra   11–19, 26, 133, 185
Hisshion, Maria   86
Hockenhull, Susan   272–9
Hollin Brow Knoll   18
Holt, Dr James   62
Holt, Ken   285
Home Office   148
Horan, Chief Superintendent Charles   138, 147
Hughes, Anthony   109–13, 122
Hughes, David   227
Hulme, Cardinal Basil   151
Human Fertilization and Embryology Act (1990)   153
Hungerford, Hampshire   255
Hyde, Greater Manchester   207

immigration   167–8
IRA (Irish Republican Army)   90, 193, 194–5, 197
Isle of Man (Summerland entertainment complex, Douglas)   281–8
Isle of Man Local Government Board   284

Jack the Ripper   5

Jackson, Graham 217, 219
Jamaica 172, 173
James (son of Maureen Bradbury) 51, 62, 66–7, 68
Jaycock, Jeffrey 120, 122
Jebb, Ian 272–6
John Paul II, Pope 151
Johnson, Susan 185
Johnson, 'White' Tony 183–5, 190
Johnson, Winnie 16, 185
Johnstone, Marty ('Mr Asia') 79–90
'Jones' family of Haslingden 303–9
Joynson, David 299–300
Joynson, Robert 300–303
Jupp, Mr Justice 242, 243
juries 187, 188
'justifiable homicide' 151

Keenan, Fr Maurice 115
Kelly, Mark 120, 122
Kendray, near Barnsley 115
Khan, Saadat 246–7
Khan, Younis 247
Kilbride, John 13, 15, 16, 22, 23
Kilu, Sabbir Kassam 311–18
King, Dr Martin Luther 170
Kingston, Jamaica 173

Lamb, Stephen 259
Lambert, Wayne 260–63
Lancashire CID vii, 311
Lancashire Police 89
    Underwater Search Unit 81
Lancaster 96
Lancaster Crown Court 87
Lane, Lord 271
laparoscope 102–3, 105
Lawler, Dr Bill 36
Leek, Staffordshire 277
Lees, Clifford 122, 123, 125
Leicester 318
Leighton Hospital 251
Lewis, 'Pommy' Harry 86
Lightbowne Hotel 140, 141
Lindow Common, Wilmslow, Cheshire 315
Lindow Pete 315
Little Budworth, Cheshire 156
Little Lever, Bolton 189
Liverpool 120, 330
Liverpool Crown Court 119, 239, 270, 317
Longford, Lord 15

Longsight, Manchester 154
Longsight police station, Manchester 176
Lord, Alan 325, 326, 328, 330–32
Lorrence, Dr Lorraine 208
Los Angeles, South Central 170–71, 172, 177
Luckhurst, Robin 156, 157
Lyons, Carlton 247–9

Macclesfield, Cheshire 272, 276, 277
McDougall, Samuel 189–90
McLennon, 'Mother' Mac 51
McLure, Professor John 36
Maher, Andrew 88, 89
Malcolm X (Malcolm Little) 170
Manchester 96, 135, 145, 161–6, 171, 187, 239, 260, 288
Manchester Airport disaster (Flight KT 328) 29–41, 281
Manchester CID 63, 147
Manchester coroner's court 57
Manchester Crown Court 134, 179, 188, 225, 245, 263, 328, 331
Manchester Evening News 18
Manchester Fire Brigade 289, 290, 293–6
Manchester mortuary 36, 139, 235, 241, 243, 261, 326
Manchester Museum 315
Manchester Royal Infirmary 244
Manchester University 315
Mandela, Nelson 170
Manson, Charles 55–6
Mantell, Mr Justice 332
Marlborough Mill 145
Marsh, Christine viii–x
Marshall, Herbert 250–53
Mary Rose (flagship) 24
Mashiter, Dr Karen 23
Meerbrook, Staffordshire 277
Mental Health Act 109
Mere Golf and Country Club, near Knutsford 93
Metropolitan Police forensic laboratory 197
Midas, King 315
Middleton mortuary, G.M. 95
Millin, Wayne 232–3
Millington, Dean 263
Moors Murderers *see* Brady, Ian; Hindley, Myra
Moreton, Wirral 197

Index

Morland, Mr Justice   263
Mosoph, Sharon   144–6
Moss Side, Manchester   161, 166–7,
      171–7, 236, 237
   gang culture case studies   178–91
Moston Brook High School   137
Mother Mac's pub murders, Manchester
      51–69
Mounsey, Detective Chief Superintendent
      Joe   vii–x
'Mr Asia' (Marty Johnstone)   79–90
murderer's appearance   55–7
Murray House, China Lane, Manchester
      293–7

Neave, Richard   315–18
New Lodge, Belfast   194
New Moston, Manchester   136
New Reno Club, Manchester   239
New South Wales   86
New York   170, 172, 177
News of the World   193, 195–6
Newton Heath, G.M.   140
Nightingale Inn, Bolton   269
Nile Club, Manchester   239–40, 241,
      243, 245
Noble's Hospital, Isle of Man   287
North, Bryan   25
North Manchester General Hospital   36
North-Western Science Laboratory,
      Chorley   90
Northenden, Manchester   110
Northern Nigeria   96
Northern Punch Bureau   293
Nottingham Motor Engineering company,
      Manchester 247
Nwagbara, Sunday 'Sunny'   240–42

O'Brien, PC David   116–17
O'Brien, Stanley   135–6
Offerton, Stockport   73
Old Bailey, London   131
Old Trafford, Manchester 247
Oldfield pub   196
Oldham, Lancashire   102, 222
Oldham and District General Hospital
      48, 154
Oldham group of hospitals   96
Oldham mortuary   22, 113, 224
Oldham Royal Infirmary   vii, viii
Ollard, Greg   86
Openshaw, Manchester   194
Ordsall, Salford   331

Organization, The   87, 88, 89, 91
Oroglass   282–3, 284, 287
Oxton, Wirral, Cheshire   215

Pack Horse Hotel, Bolton   144–5
Pankhania, Mansukhlal   188–9, 190
Parhatka, Sandra   185–7, 190
Park Hospital, Davyhulme, G.M.   viii,
      248
Parkhurst Jail, Isle of Wight   90
pathology, role of   95–6
Penny Black pub, Cheetham Hill,
      Manchester   183
Peppermint Place club, Blackburn   228,
      230
Percival, Joan   155–7
Philip of Macedon   315
police
   arming   107–8
   death of policemen   107, 108–9,
      113–15, 117–19, 120–25
Police Gazette   253
Polson, Professor Harry   22
Poplar Street Primary School, Ashton-
      under-Lyne   207–8
post-mortem   3–7
Prestbury, Cheshire   271–2
Preston Crown Court   125, 128–9, 308
Preston Royal Infirmary   82
Price, Jack, QC   206
'pro-life' lobby   158, 159
Proverbs, Henderson   178, 179–81, 183,
      190
Puljik, Vinko, Archbishop of Sarajevo
      151

Queen's Park Hospital, Blackburn   228

racism   169–72, 256–63
Railway pub, Farnworth   270
Reade, Amos   9, 10, 12, 21
Reade, Joan   9, 10, 12, 21
Reade, Paul   21
Reade, Pauline   9–14, 16, 17, 18, 20–22
   autopsy   23–7, 185
Ridgway, Detective Superintendent Jack
      62–3, 65
Risley prison, Warrington   215
River Orin see Flight KT 328 disaster
      (Manchester Airport)
Rochdale, Lancashire   159, 257, 260
Rossendale public mortuary   307
Rothwell, Geoffrey   94

Royal Air Force (RAF) 30, 33, 36, 38, 40
Royal Liverpool Hospital 120
Royal Preston Hospital 123
Russell, Mr Justice 328
Ryan, Michael 238–9, 246, 255
Rye, Sydney, Australia 87

Saddleworth, near Oldham 322
Saddleworth Moor 12, 15, 16, 18–21, 26, 185
Saddleworth mortuary 22
St Paul's, Bristol 167
Scott, James Alexander 266–70
Sheffield 320
Sheffield Children's Hospital 204
Shell Chemicals, Carrington 24
Sills, Dr John 205–6
Sinclair, Alexander 83–7, 89, 90, 91
Sinclair, Jarrod 91
Sindall, Diane 217–22
Skala, Wanda 140–42, 144, 146
Skuse, Frank 286
Smith, Winifred 226–7
Spinner's Arms pub, Hulme 179
Stanley, Benji 176
Steel, David (later Sir David) 152, 153
Stepping Hill Hospital, Stockport 235
Steptoe, Patrick 102–6
Stewart, Janet Lesley 134, 136–40, 146–7
Stewart, Julian 'Turbo' 175
Stockport, G.M. 145
Strangeways Jail, Manchester 90
    riot (1990) 328–31
Sullivan, Peter 215–17, 221
Summerfield, Donald 296
Summerland entertainment complex,
    Douglas, Isle of Man 281–8
Sutcliffe, Peter (the Yorkshire Ripper)
    55–6, 131–2, 133, 255
Sydney Airport 86
Sydney Harbour 86

Tameside, G.M. 259
Tameside Borough Council 208
Tameside Hospital, Ashton-under-Lyne 202
Tarporley War Memorial Hospital,
    Cheshire 155, 157
Tate, Sharon 56
Taylor, Geoffrey 223, 225
Taylor, Lynne 222–5

Terrington, Captain Peter 30–31
'test tube' babies 102–6, 158
thalidomide 153
Theilman, Julie 86
Tiller, Jackie 319–22, 324
time of death 4
Topping, Chief Superintendent Peter
    13–19, 24, 26
Toxteth, Liverpool 167
Trafford Park, Manchester 49
Tuinol 71

Ulster 109, 194, 195
Urmston Police Station vii
Usher, Dr Alan 278

Valance, Philip, QC 178–9
Variend, Dr S. 204–5, 209
video cameras 146
VO15 unit 176

Waddington, David, QC 128
Walker, Peter 178–9
Walsh, David 115, 275–80
Walsh, Linda 276
Werneth, Oldham 222
West Didsbury, Greater Manchester 237
West Park Hospital, Macclesfield 273
Whalley Range, Manchester 161
Whitbread Brewery 51–2, 54, 64, 67
White, Derek 328–30, 331–2
Whitwell, Dr Helen 209, 210
Williams, Chief Superintendent Gerald 279
Williams and Glyn's Bank, Prestbury
    272–3, 276, 279
Wilmslow, Cheshire 24
Wilson, Douglas 87
Wilson, Isobel 87
Withington, Manchester 261
Withington Hospital, Manchester 36, 320
Woodcock, Dr R. Cyril 141, 146
Woodward, PC Ian 122–5
Woolworth's store, Piccadilly Gardens,
    Manchester 288–93
Worsley, G.M. 250
Wrightson, Dr Phillip 199, 200, 210–11
    Head Injuries – the Facts 199

Yardie gangs 172, 173
Yorkshire Ripper *see* Sutcliffe Peter